Nature's
Goldmine

Other Books by Dr. Allan C. Somersall

Breakthrough In Cell-Defense
with Dr. Gustavo Bounous

Your Very Good Health: 101 Healthy Lifestyle Choices

A Passion For Living: The Art of Real Success

Your Evolution to YES!

Understanding The Evolution of YES!

Evolutionary Tales by Dr. YES!

Nature's Goldmine

Harvesting
MIRACLE INGREDIENTS
from MILK

Allan C. Somersall, Ph.D., M.D.

Author of the Bestselling Book
'Breakthrough In Cell-Defense'

GOLDENeight Publishers
Toronto * Atlanta

Copyright© 2001 by Allan Somersall, GOLDENeight Publishers
Cover Design: Cynthia Koelsch Design

Printed in Canada

Library of Congress Cataloging-in-Publication Data
ISBN # 1-890412-89-9
Includes references and index

Nature's Goldmine ... Harvesting Miracle Ingredients from Milk /
Allan C. Somersall - E-mail: doctor@doctoryes.net

10 9 8 7 6 5 4 3 2   1

Published By:
GOLDENeight Publishers
2-3415 Dixie Road, Suite: 538
Mississauga, Ontario CANADA L4Y 2B1
Offices in Canada and the United States
1-800-501-8516
www.goldeneightbooks.com
E-Mail: goldeneightbooks@aol.com

*Dedicated
to
my brother,
Terry*

ACKNOWLEDGEMENTS

The author is indebted to a number of people who made valuable contribution to this book:

to Chuck Roberts, for his original proposal;

to Carolina Loren, for her diligent and extensive research, preparing the manuscript and tireless continuous editing;

to Irene Lamour and colleagues at INGREDIA for the original work on Chapter IX and useful additional comments;

to Dr. Stephen Petrosino,Nutritionist, for major input to Chapter X;

to a mentor, Dr. Gustavo Bounous for review and valuable comments;

to Bev Livingston for his personal tour of a modern dairy farm;

to Cynthia Koelsch for the original cover design;

to Kathryn Stephens at Immunotec Research & Michelle Galateau at Advitech Solutions, for effective communications;

to my dear family, for their patience, support and encouragement; and finally,

to my publisher GOLDENeight, for championing the book and guiding it through to completion.

To all of you, I am most grateful, for without such a formidable support cast, this book would not be a reality. In the end, all the shortcomings are mine.

Allan Somersall, Ph.D., M.D.

DISCLAIMER STATEMENT

This book is designed to provide general information to the public at large. Nothing herein is intended to advise or encourage the reader to practice any form of self-diagnosis or treatment. Medical problems should always be addressed by competent healthcare professionals on an individual basis. Therefore, this is not a medical prescription or even a suggested first point of reference. Nutritional and health needs vary from person to person, depending on such factors as age, sex, health status and total lifestyle.

TABLE OF CONTENTS

INTRODUCTION

Every modern bookstore in North America has a section devoted to Health. Browsing through the books on these shelves quickly reveals a novel paradox. At the dawn of this new millenium, one would imagine that the public at large would be in praise of all the outstanding achievements of science and medicine in the last century. Clearly, we have improved the diagnostic and therapeutic capabilities, perhaps orders of magnitude during that time. But surprisingly, the lay press and an increasing number of health professionals have turned south and the consuming public, for a variety of reasons, is in search of alternative approaches to health care.

Hardly a day goes by that I do not hear a patient or some acquaintance or other, expressing the frustration of conflicting information coming from every interest group in the health and medicine arena. What was promoted yesterday as being so 'good for you' and 'an ideal lifestyle choice for your family', is losing favor today and may be subject to some critical report that warns the consumer to 'beware'. We are increasingly flooded with information and much misinformation in the area of self-help and health responsibility, thereby making sensible informed choices most difficult.

Amidst the confusion, the public is losing trust because one hardly knows whom to trust. Even traditional authority figures have lost their credibility in the minds of consumers because there is so much diversity of opinion and there is so much compromise in the name of political correctness and media sensation. Claims are constantly being neutralized by counter-claims.

That's why I have taken such delight in writing this book. It is addressed directly to the searching consumer who wants real answers, not convenient sound-bites or quick-fixes. The subject is addressed right at the interface of nature and science. The simple thesis is that only the very best that nature affords, subjected to the best scrutiny that science allows, can provide the best avenues to optimum health and wellness. Nature's goldmine is a surprising but revealing source.

In Part One, **Making the Link**, we first take a brief but panoramic view of the Alternative Medicine arena. We survey the so-called complementary health professions, techniques and therapies that are gaining increasing popularity. That overview prompts the question which arises if one goes back to the basics of nature: Whatever became of milk? That immediately introduces a controversy. Behind all the dairy industry's promotional hype and public relations strategy, is cow's milk really a healthy nutritional panacea ... or could it be a disguised poison? Only good science could provide real answers. Hence, a call is made to apply the proven scientific method as we explore nature's goldmine.

Defending the Body, in Part Two, addresses a central theme of all Wellness advocates -- improving the immune system, in real terms. A new paradigm is introduced to focus on cell-defense and the role of the master intracellular antioxidant, glutathione. The serendipitous discovery in Canada of unique whey proteins in nature's goldmine, which deliver the rate-limiting precursor for GSH synthesis, provides a safe, effective and convenient handle that promises to accelerate the glutathione revolution. It demands that both researchers and consumers rethink health and medicine and the role of glutathione and cell-defense in both prevention and management of disease.

In Part Three, **Calming the Mind**, we report another major find that relates to the most common mental condition in contemporary industralized society - anxiety. After a review of mental illness and anxiety in particular, we trace the systematic discovery in France of the active peptide ingredient buried in nature's goldmine, that attaches to the benzodiazepine-type receptor for the most prevalent inhibitory neurotransmitter in the brain, GABA. It has such a calming effect that it may be accurately designated as 'nature's tranquilizing peptide.'

Finally in Part Four, **Taking home Gold**, we get to the popular notion of calcium as synonymous with milk and vice versa, only to conclude that modern technology affords the pure milk calcium from nature's goldmine without any of the downsides of whole milk consumption.

As the reader, you can make your own choices, informed by just the facts. Don't miss out on the tour to a modern dairy farm in Chapter Eleven. It is a breath of fresh air and an experience of nature to replace the insanity of the metropolis. But in the end, you must cultivate good nutritional habits and practice a lifestyle of coping strategies that will allow you to defend your body from within your cells, and to calm your mind effectively.

Take full advantage therefore, of the harvested ingredients of nature's goldmine, and do enjoy the best of health.

Go for the Gold,
Allan Somersall, Ph.D., M.D.

PART
1

MAKING
THE
LINK

Chapter One

BACK TO NATURE
A peek into the Alternative Medicine Arena

As this generation enters the twenty first century, a few characteristics define the mid-life population wave as much as the search for Wellness. We're on a mission to enjoy the best of life and to preserve our health with all the vigor and virility that our genes will allow. We've declared war on cancer, heart disease and AIDS. We're making lifestyle changes in record numbers and we're prepared to defend our health rights by any means necessary. We're going to do all we can to stay healthy and young, and to look like it. If the good life is this good, then it is worth prolonging to the ultimate state that nature and science will allow. After all, in our contemporary space and times, the pursuit of happiness means searching for the combined product of both the quality and the quantity of life.

Enter Rick and Celeste –
They are baby boomers, living in booming times. They belong to this electronic generation obsessed with youth, freedom and productivity. They have it all, but live in fear of losing it all, as the pace of change accelerates and the brevity and uncertainty of life confronts their affluence and vitality.

So, this morning is no different. While their adolescent kids are still asleep, Rick and Celeste are up at the crack of dawn. They go jogging along their usual three kilometer route as the sun comes up to greet them in the neighborhood park. Daylight Saving Time allows them to enjoy the great outdoors. And in the winter, they take turns to push themselves on the exercise bike in their basement. In either case, it is now a sacred ritual. They bought into Dr. Cooper's aerobics agenda and there's no stopping them.

After washing up, it's down to a breakfast fare of hot oatmeal or muesli; fruit or juice; whole wheat pastry or granola bars, and herbal tea. Rick scans the morning paper and soon steers his BMW into rush hour traffic to his downtown office. He is a computer sales-man. Celeste is an interior decorator and works from her home office. She too is internet-savvy and keeps up with what's new on the 'health and wellness' front.

Rick and Celeste are fortunately still in good health. Now in their forties, they are anxious to keep it that way. Periodic health exams with their physicians are a must, but so also are their regular visits to their other health care providers. Rick is an avid squash player and is frequently at the chiropractor's office for adjustments to ease his aching back. Celeste swears that her weekly massage is therapeutic for both mind and body.

Their two boys are also in fine health now, active in sports and academically motivated. The younger one was home-birthed and the parents are still convinced that there's something special about him. When he was younger, he suffered from recurrent ear infections and endured several courses of antibiotics. Eventually, he was seen by an acupuncturist and to this day, the parents are convinced that those fine needles solved his problem. The older boy had a similar story with recurrent asthma – until he saw a herbalist who designed a concoction of herbal remedies that seemed to do the trick.

Don't try telling these yuppie parents that those are coinciden-tal anecdotes. They refuse to accept any suggestion that these were the natural courses of either condition. They judge by results. They be-lieve that medical doctors don't have all the answers. They read widely and have a keen interest in natural remedies and all aspects of comple-mentary medicine.

Rick and Celeste are products of their generation.

It is most ironic that at the end of "the Medical Century", with its dramatic advances in orthodox diagnostic and treatment protocols, we enter this new century with a renewed focus on *alternative* and *complementary* healing arts. Could it really be that as MRI scanners and gene manipulation techniques are becoming more commonplace, many people are now looking to iridologists for their clinical diagnosis and to colonic treatments as a panacea for what ails them?

The western world has applied all the sophistication of modern science and its understanding of the human frame to convert the *art* of medicine into a true *science*. And there are so many triumphs and accomplishments to prove it. From organ transplants and laser surgery, to brain mapping or anti-retroviral cocktails, we have clearly entered a new era of human existence.

But chronic degenerative problems remain. We are all getting older and many debilitating conditions are still as prevalent as ever. We're demanding more and more. We're looking for answers and sometimes in all the wrong places.

THE WELLNESS MOVEMENT

Perhaps the greatest shift in public demands and expectations in recent time has been the increasing influence of the so-called Wellness Movement. Popularized by media personalities and best-selling authors, the focus on health – on feeling good and looking good – and the anticipated counter-current to advances in modern medicine have been taking hold.

Yes, refusing to accept the frailty of the human condition and the limitations of modern medicine, there has been a growing movement to rediscover the so-called *wisdom of the ages*. It has been a step backward in time, but protagonists would argue that it has also been a step forward in outlook ... a philosophical shift in the understanding of mind-body-nature interactions. It reflects a desire to harness more than the sum of the parts into which science now dissects the human body. Hence, a new vocabulary. It is the emergence of *whole-istic* healthcare. *Whole-istic* or *holistic* healthcare covers the wide range of treatment options that are generally not a part of conventional medical practice. These traditional options are usually not viewed as *alternatives*, but as *complements* intended to boost one's potential for health and recovery. They cannot compete with any of the emergency procedures, or the indispensable therapeutics, or the appropriate surgical interventions of conventional *allopathic* medicine. But they are heralded as being uniquely suited for the preservation and promotion of health and wellness. In addition, there are claims of their healing potential for many common and chronic ailments that truly affect one's quality of life. For many, the *natural* alternative is the first option. They contend that doctors are trained and oriented towards illness and acute care and therefore should probably be the last resort in the pursuit of wellness.

But then, Wellness takes on a philosophical significance. The belief that the mind influences the body and that the body, in turn, has an impact on the mind, is a key element in the philosophy of almost all *alternative* or *complementary* care. As a result, this approach focuses on the health needs of the *whole person*. Practitioners strive to be aware of their *clients'* health from the different perspectives: physical, emotional, nutritional, environmental and spiritual factors are all considered. The emphasis is always on the body's (otherwise described as nature's) ability to *heal itself* with the help of natural, non-invasive therapies which they proclaim are often effective and without harmful side effects.

Complementary care promotes the education of its clients since it often necessitates positive lifestyle changes. Practitioners work in *partnership* with their clients, teaching them novel ideas but more importantly, motivating them toward better health and helping to strengthen the *internal healing potential* of each individual. The goal is to restore *balance* and *harmony* of mind and body. It is to put the clients' wellbeing into their own hands so that they can become active participants in their own recovery and/or health maintenance.

Although many in the traditional medical community continue to debunk these ideas and the treatments that are advocated by the Wellness gurus, the public clearly does not agree. Instead most people seem to have embraced Alternative Medicine as part of their personal health care regimen. Rick and Celeste are more the rule than the exception today. A study in the *Journal of the American Medical Association (JAMA)* recently indicated that Americans now visit Alternative care providers much more often than traditional physicians, and the numbers are increasing. In 1997, Americans spent an estimated $27 billion on visits to alternative practitioners, a 45 percent increase over 1990. And most of that was out of their own pockets directly.

People have been alienated from an increasingly impersonal

health care system. Traditional medicine is clearly recognized for its emergency drama and heroics. But it is also seen as expensive, impersonal and in the end, not all that effective at promoting health, but rather at just treating symptomatic illness. On the other hand, alternative therapists are perceived as more attentive, responsive and willing to give the patient a role in their treatment and its outcome.

It seems apparent then, that we are seeking long-term health care, not quick-fix cures. We want more prevention and less pills. Most of all, we want to feel cared for as persons. We are willing to take a chance on the outcome of the tried but yet unproven modalities that offer hope and caring, and even to pay out of our own pockets.

From all appearance, we seem to be heading to a great divide. It's nature *or* science. But then our health may be put at risk.

Much of the subject matter in later chapters of this book will refer to the relationship of nature, science and health as we attempt to make the connection with one common natural source. That will become an indispensable link. So here we begin with *nature* and what is becoming more popular with the natural approach to health and even disease. Later we will pick up *science* and have them court into marriage, and give birth to better *health*.

What follows next then, is a brief synopsis for the uninitiated of the more common *alternative* or *complementary* healing approaches that have gained a foothold in the growing Wellness Movement in the Western world. First, we'll take a brief look at the major alternative healthcare **professions** that have earned respectability. Then we shall consider some critical therapeutic **techniques** in common practice in the Wellness community. Finally, in this chapter, we shall summarize the known characteristics of the nutritional and other **therapies** to lay the foundation for the major thrust of this book. After this panoramic tour, we will find that nature's biggest goldmine for healthy body and healthy mind has indeed been very present and yet remains untapped.

But there is good news to follow later.

NATURAL HEALING PROFESSIONS

In the interest of time and space, one could not do justice to the natural healing professions in this brief overview. All we can do is to set the stage for what is to follow, as we explore the exciting interface, first of nature and then of science.

Naturopathy

Naturopathy is best explained through its philosophies which can be stated in three common assertions.

1. The human body has the ability to heal itself;
2. Symptoms are not part of a disease, but are signs that the body is working to eliminate toxins;
3. A person should be treated as a whole, taking into account physical, psychological or emotional, and genetic factors.

This approach is not a single medical theory developed by any one person, but rather it is a combination of healing approaches drawn from various parts of the world. Naturopathy is, in fact, the modern umbrella profession of Alternative Medicine and includes wisdom from the medicines of ancient Greek, Chinese, Indian and Native American cultures.

Naturopathic doctors (with the N.D. degree) believe in the healing power of nature, and treat patients by 'seeking to restore overall health rather than suppressing a few key symptoms'. Then they seek to apply treatments that work in alliance with the so-called *natural* healing mechanisms of the body rather than against them.

Naturopathic physicians are less focused on individual organ systems and differential diagnoses. They work with the patient to determine a generalized cause of the presenting illness, and apply their therapies in a way to restore overall health. They may at times use palliative or symptomatic treatments, but only in the context of overall health restoration.

Homeopathy

Homeopathy is a system of medicine which also claims to assist the natural tendency of the body to heal itself. It is based on the principle of "like curing like" formulated in 1790 by Dr. Samuel

Hahnemann. He found that substances of plant, mineral, or animal origin, given to a healthy person in repeated doses can cause that person to become ill in a specific way by producing quite unique symptoms. More importantly, the same substance (in an extremely small dose) could cure a sick person with a similar set of naturally occurring symptoms. Hahnemann found that the medicines became more effective if they were shaken (potentized) and diluted. This paradoxical effect of increased effectiveness with less substance has never been explained, and is one of the major stumbling blocks that conventional medical thinkers have in relation to homeopathy.

Today, the most common form of homeopathic medicines are tiny pills that dissolve when placed under the tongue. They are made from all-natural substances, including plants, roots, and minerals. It is believed that these substances act like booster cables, stimulating the body's own healing response, whatever that maybe. The necessary strength and dosage amount is specific to each person being treated.

Such individualization begs the question, but in the absence of adequate standardized clinical trials, it is difficult to see the relevance of homeopathy for any major illness today.

Osteopathy

Doctors of Osteopathic Medicine (with the D.O. degree) are fully licensed and recognized healthcare providers who stress the *unity of all body systems.* They focus on the musculoskeletal system and also emphasize holistic medicine, proper nutrition and environmental factors. They bring a hands-on approach to medicine and view palpation and manipulation as aids to the diagnosis and treatment of various illnesses. They recognize the close relationship between body structure and organ functioning, and also consider the patient's mental and emotional status. In addition, the D.O. pays attention to the relationship of the patient to his or her home environment, job and other factors that affect health. Some would argue that it was the D.O.'s who pioneered the concept of "Wellness" more than 100 years ago. In today's terms, personal health risks - such as smoking, high blood pressure, excessive cholesterol levels, stress and other life-style factors – are evaluated for each individual. In coordination with appropriate medical treatments, the osteopath acts as a teacher and guide to help patients take more responsibility for their own health and make necessary changes. By combining unique osteopathic principles with traditional diagnostic and therapeutic procedures, D.O.'s offer a balanced system of healthcare to both prevent and cure disease. It is a type of practice designed for the *Wellness* Age.

Chiropractic

Chiropractic is a *natural* method of healing which it is claimed utilizes the body's own recuperative powers. The chiropractic system is based on the belief that a strong, agile, and aligned spine is the key to good health. And that is so for a particular reason. Only when the body is receiving 100% of the central nervous system's impulses can it operate at its 100% capacity. When interference occurs and the nerve energy is blocked whatever healing factors that nerve supplies cannot function at their full potential. Since the body receives and transmits messages to the brain via the 33 pairs of spinal nerves which are housed within the spine, perfect alignment is critical.

In principle, therefore, interference most often occurs when a vertebra (segment of the spine) becomes misaligned with the surrounding bones, causing irritation to soft tissue and most importantly, to the nerves. The nerves can become entrapped, compressed or pinched. Dysfunction results, which according to the chiropractic theory, results in a lowered resistance to infection and disease in the areas of the body supplied by the particular nerves. Trauma, repetitive injury (such as occupational lifting), poor posture and congenital problems account for a majority of incidences of misalignment (and therefore, illness). It is the job of the Chiropractor (with the D.C. degree) to find the cause of the interference of nerve transmission and correct it. The chiropractor manipulates and makes adjustments to the spine. Then with the backbone in its proper position, the nervous system is now free to send out the necessary signals for the human body to function normally.

Based on the limited number of clinical trials, the most reliable results are for the relief of straightforward musculo-skeletal symptomatology or nerve irritation leading principally to pain and/or weakness. A major problem can arise if there is any aggressive effort to extend the indications for spinal manipulation to conditions that clearly warrant only pharmaceutical or surgical intervention. Most chiropractors have sought to broaden their otherwise narrow sphere of practice by including dietary advice and nutritional counseling, rehabilitative exercises, massage and job-related body mechanics. Many have added their own special lifestyle or wholistic interests. They tend to practice 'chiropractic-Plus.'

NATURAL HEALING TECHNIQUES

Several healing techniques outside the normal practice of allopathic medicine go back hundreds of years. Some have their origins in philosophy as much as in practical experience, but what they all do have in common is the active intervention with the patient or client. Healthcare is indeed a therapeutic relationship as much as it is something to ingest or consume. More and more, the public in the Western World is demanding time and attention from those who would look after their bodies and their health. No longer will "take this pill and call me in the morning" have any place in healthcare. No more will a prescription pad substitute for a helpful dialogue or therapeutic touch. As we pointed out, much of the appeal of the *alternative* and *complementary* practitioners derives from their tendency to active intervention and care. We saw this in the few professions that we just outlined and we will see it again in the natural healing techniques which we discuss briefly below, as we continue to explore the interface with *nature*.

Acupuncture

Acupuncture is based on the belief that health is maintained by an orderly flow of universal life energy called *Qi (Chi)* through a complex system of meridian pathways in the body. Illness and pain result when the flow of *Qi* is blocked. This can be corrected by inserting acupuncture needles at specific sites (points) where appropriate meridians are in close contact with the surface of the body.

A number of clinical trials have established the value of this technique although the precise mechanism of action is still debated by the researchers in this field. The hallmark benefit that has been established is in analgesia – chronic pain relief. But many common physical disorders and complaints are believed to stem from blocked energy channels.

The acupuncture needles vary. The procedure can sometimes be enhanced by heat (moxibustion) and/or electricity. Mastering the proper technique for needle insertion and knowing where and how to do this, requires lengthy training and experience. It is also important to detect exactly when the area of blockage has been reached.

The technique is now well established in North America today and is probably here to stay. About 13 million Americans have already turned to acupuncture, the majority of whom are treated by trained physicians.

Magnet Therapy

A 4000 year old Chinese medical text describes how lodestones applied to acupuncture points could relieve pain by increasing the flow of *Qi(Chi)* energy to certain parts of the body. In the middle of the 18th century, magnet mania swept through Europe, largely due to Franz Anton Mesmer, a charismatic physician who reported miraculous cures. Mesmer used all sorts of magnetic paraphernalia in his Parisian salon to increase the flow of his "animal magnetism," which allegedly could heal anything.

Although Mesmer was discredited, the popularity of magnets steadily soared in the U.S. By the beginning of the last century, magnetic insoles, rings, belts, girdles, caps and other apparel were sold to treat everything from athletes' feet and baldness, to menstrual cramps and impotency. Their popularity naturally declined with the advent of drugs and surgical procedures that could provide proven benefits. However, there has been a remarkable resurgence of interest in the past few years due to the explosion of enthusiasm in *Alternative Medicine*. In particular, a successful MLM company from Japan has popularized the use of magnet therapy in North America by drawing on its widespread application in Asia.

There is good evidence that permanent magnets can provide some pain relief for patients. It is estimated that magnets are used by over 100 million people worldwide, and are licensed in some countries. Placebo effects cannot be excluded. In fact, it is not clear how permanent magnets achieve their effects. The problem is that there is very little control over the manufacture and use of permanent magnets. Since they are considered to be natural products rather than medical devices, they are not subject to FDA requirements to show both efficacy and safety. The use of magnetic fields as therapy is being studied as part of a $1.2 million grant from the U.S. Office of Alternative Medicine. Double-blind studies in patients with fibromyalgia, carpal tunnel syndrome, and low back pain at medical school-affiliated centers could provide the proof necessary to obtain FDA approval for the use of magnets for pain relief.

Massage Therapy

Massage therapy is based on the principle of human touch. It is simply the practice of kneading or manipulating a person's muscles and other soft tissue with the intent of improving that individual's well-being. Its concept is instinctual; most people immediately react to injury by rubbing the traumatized area of the body. The sensation of touch is one of the oldest and best known ways to demonstrate caring and to provide comfort. So massage is a natural way of relaxing tired, sore muscles. It is probably the oldest method of alleviating pain and other symptoms of disease and promoting good health. Massage dates back three thousand years before Christ and was used by the Chinese, Japanese, Indians, Greeks and Romans to maintain a strong and healthy body to treat illness. The two best known modalities of massage are Swedish massage based on body systems. (Western tradition), and Shiatsu based on *yin/yang* meridians (Eastern orientation).

Massage is a personal service with individualized results. Doctors acknowledge the therapeutic value for musculo-skeletal and soft tissue injury, pain management and rehabilitation. In any case, it is essentially a benign procedure although there are some acute contraindications. The final benefit of any massage should be a sense of well-being, both physiological and psychological.

Reflexology

Reflexology is an ancient healing therapy based on the *theory* that there are reflex areas in the feet which anatomically correspond to all parts of the body. Stimulating these reflexes correctly can relieve tension and stress in a natural way. Practitioners advocate this therapeutic modality for a wide variety of common ailments, but the clinical indications are very vague and suspect, to say the least. However, reflexology is practiced in all parts of the world by different cultures. It has found limited acceptance in North America.

The theory goes that sediments caused by stress, tension and gravity accumulate in the foot and cause micro-crystallization. At those points, the energy flow (associate *Qi, Chi*) to some corresponding body parts is blocked. The reflexologist presumably knows how to recognize this congestion. By pressing (not massaging) with his/her fingers and thumbs, the therapist can help dissolve the microcrystals causing the congestion to re-create a positive energy flow. But that's not all. This energy flow is then believed to help the body *heal itself.*

This is a technique that again probably 'does no harm' but its real therapeutic value beyond placebo is certainly questionable.

Biofeedback

The term "biofeedback" was coined in the late 1960s to describe procedures that were used to train research subjects to alter physiological variables that normally are not controlled voluntarily. These included nerve transmission, smooth muscle tone, brain activity, blood pressure, heart rate and other bodily functions. This is the ultimate in restoring health responsibility to the individual patient by giving them conscious and deliberate control over their own bodies. It is an attempt to exploit by training a presumed brain function connecting the voluntary and involuntary control centers, just as we learn to outgrow bedwetting for example.

Biofeedback therapy (training), begins with sensitive instruments designed to measure a specific physiological process, e.g., the electrical activity of skeletal muscles. The instrument is connected to the muscle with adhesive skin sensors; it amplifies and converts the physiological response into meaningful information which is "fed back" to the patient, who then uses the information as a guide, while practicing a variety of procedures to achieve reduced muscle tension.

Today, biofeedback is a safe, non-invasive, non-pharmacological treatment sometimes used alone or as a valuable adjunct to more traditional therapies in conditions like anxiety disorders, attention deficit hyperactivity disorder (ADHD), cerebral palsy, headaches, enuresis or incontinence, motion sickness, myofascial pain, neuro-muscular pain and sleep disorders.

Hypnotherapy

If biofeedback trains the individual to take more control, hypnotherapy does the direct opposite. Hypnotherapy is an approach during which the therapist guides the client into a trance-like state called *hypnosis,* where one loses control. In the hypnotic state, the client becomes most relaxed, capable of intense concentration, and open to suggestions for change. This state can be induced through several simple techniques, among which are verbal suggestions and having the patient observe a continuously moving object.

Since the mid-fifties, the medical establishment has recognized the value and effectiveness of hypnotherapy. A growing number of physicians use hypnosis to improve their patients' physical and mental health. Hypnosis can ease childbirth, and while still rarely used as an anesthetic, it is frequently employed to make surgery and recovery more pleasant for the patient. Psychotherapists of many backgrounds include hypnotherapy in their practices. Today, it is recognized as an effective technique in the management of some psychological and psychosomatic conditions.

NUTRITIONAL THERAPIES

Of all the *natural* interventions that have become popular with all the attendant media hype and more, nutritional therapies have clearly gained the most attention. There is a constant stream of fad diets, new products, therapeutic claims, original recipes and concoctions which promise to ease one or other of our many chronic complaints.

After all, what could be more natural than eating, and it is obvious that '*we become what we eat,*' as Adelle Davis was apt to point out. Nutrition then, is fundamental to well-being and generally is a common denominator in every physical condition. Needless to say, this fact has become more than just a 'mantra' to all the Wellness advocates. It is perceived by some to be the panacea we've all neglected. If we only knew our bodies better, and fed them as we should, we would experience robust health and long life.

But not quite so fast.

Nutrition is a science – a relatively young science indeed. It is the series of processes by which any living organism takes in and assimilates food for producing energy, promoting growth, combating infection, replacing worn or injured tissues, and thinking. Without the proper nutrients, humans do cause damage to the body and impair the body's normal functioning. Proper nutrition is different for each person, varying with a person's state of health, digestive tract, physical environment, body composition and activity level. Good nutrition certainly goes beyond the Food and Drug Administration's RDA formulae for basic existence. Optimal nutrition should provide people with the ability to optimize their lives, while offering a strong defense against degenerative disease. As such, it should strengthen the immune system and aid in recuperation in the face of any illness.

Many studies have now established the central role of nutrition in both the origin, management and prognosis of many major and minor illnesses. Dieticians and nutritionists have become knowledgeable in analyzing dietary intake and designing appropriate diets for optimum benefits in both health and disease. The most recent edition of the comprehensive textbook 'Modern Nutrition in Health and Disease', (Lippincott, Williams & Wilkins, 1999) has over 1900 pages of practical information. Government agencies have developed specific recommendations for the daily intake of all essential nutrients. The term essential underlines the importance of each element in the diet and characteristic diseases are associated with each nutrient deficiency.

The dieticians have defined the various classes of foods: proteins (amino acids), carbohydrates (starches), fats (some essential), vitamins (water- and fat-soluble), minerals (macro-and micro-), fiber (soluble and insoluble), and finally, water. They have taught us how to have an adequate diet (minimum calories to supply energy/fuel) and a balanced diet (different ratios of each category and subcategory). They have given us the Food Pyramid as a guide. They have warned us against the dangers of high fat and cholesterol. They have underlined the importance of high fiber and the value of fruits and vegetables. They have cursed the successful promotion of fast, convenient junk foods. They have criticized the fad-diets with the associated weight-loss pendulum.

But that is just the beginning. They did not go far enough. The Wellness disciples have an implicit faith in the power of natural food to empower the body to protect and even to heal itself. They are constantly seeking to exploit some new benefit from a traditional food or novel food supplement. And there are an increasing number to choose from.

Vitamin Supplementation

Repeated dietary surveys in the US and Canada have consistently shown inadequacies in vitamin intake in the typical diet. Consumers in any case, are leading the statisticians. They are swallowing vitamins, minerals and herbal supplements in unprecedented numbers to ward off illness, prolong their lives and hopefully, maintain youthful looks and energy.

According to *The Globe and Mail, Toronto,* the most recent Angus Reid telephone survey across Canada in early 2000 found that in the previous month, two out of three adult Canadians ages 18 to 65 had taken some form of nutritional supplement – from glucosamine for arthritic joints to antioxidant vitamins for healthier skin. The supplement market in Canada is now estimated at $1.8 billion a year (in the U.S., $15-20 billion). The use of vitamins is the most popular among these supplement users (60 percent in the survey), but the use of herbal supplements is growing most dramatically. Vitamins and herbal supplements are readily available over the counter in drugstores, pharmacies and health food stores, as well as by direct marketing and now e-commerce. U.S. sales of megavitamins alone rose from $0.9 billion in 1990 to $3.3 billion in 1997. As discretionary items, they do much better in a strong economy.

Unfortunately, the increased interest in these health products has a downside. Two thirds of these consumers tend to leave their doctors out of the loop, since they presume the doctors are ill-informed about supplements and are often critical. The problem is that some natural health products have active ingredients that can interact adversely with prescription medications and sometimes with each other. Indications are that younger doctors are now following their patients lead and are struggling to catch up. That's a hopeful trend. A new *Natural Medicines Comprehensive Database* (Therapeutic Research Faculty, Stockton, CA., 1999) has recently become available to physicians.

Most vitamins were discovered by studying the clinical diseases associated with their deficiencies such as scurvy, pellagra, pernicious anemia, and so on. Both water-soluble vitamins (a complex of B's and C) and fat-soluble vitamins (A, D, E and K) have long since been characterized, synthesized and commercialized. Many doctors have linked the dietary intake of individual vitamins with clinical implications for prevention and management of corresponding illnesses. The orthodox health care establishment has still held that vitamin supplementation is not generally indicated (with absence of disease) and have advocated simple diets rich in fruits and vegetables. But what are they afraid of? Cases of vitamin toxicity usually reflect only the accidental exploration by small children at home or the extreme behavior associated with mental illness. The argument of wasting money in expensive urine is scarcely relevant with the explosive market for junk food. The fear that pill-popping would encourage poor-diets has also proven unwarranted, since all studies agree that vitamin users have clearly the best diets in society.

In any case, millions of North Americans have seen the consummate wisdom of daily vitamin supplementation and have now cultivated this as a lifestyle habit. The Wellness buffs have gone beyond that to learn the value of different vitamins so that they can appropriately choose their unique supplement cocktail. The focus has recently been on the anti-oxidant vitamins A, C and E. These have particularly been associated with the fight against cancer, cholesterol, cataracts and many other prevalent clinical conditions. Individual B vitamins have also become popular now that a lack of folic acid in pregnancy, for example, has been associated with neural tube defects. Vitamin sales through drug stores, pharmacies, health food stores and direct marketing, have become a billion-dollar industry.

In a word, the value of vitamin supplementation has been justified and in any case, the practice is here to stay.

Organ Extracts

It may seem somewhat strange, at least to the analytical mind, that another alternative health approach involves ingesting extracts from animal organs and glands with the hope that these would somehow support and revitalize human organs and glands.

Advanced medical research has recently sought to surgically transplant healthy active cells into specific organs to hopefully enhance or restore the production of some essential hormones. For example, early successful transplants of islet cells of the pancreas have proven effective for increased insulin production in diabetics, and similarly, transplant of dopamine producing brain cells has recently shown promise for Parkinsonian disease management. Complete organ transplant is now an almost routine surgical procedure under the right conditions for heart, lung, kidney, liver, etc., in end-stage disease. Bone marrow transplants, corneal transplants and skin grafts have been around for a long time.

But all this is unrelated to the proposed *alternative* protocol of ingesting animal extracts. These extracts consist of compositions of varying quality and purity. Some are bioactive enzymes or nucleoproteins, while others are whole organ preparations. Some extracts are predigested for easy assimilation. For example, liquid liver extract is a specific fraction of beef liver, rich in nutrients but no fat or cholesterol, which is broken down into small chains of amino acids to provide a highly concentrated complex readily absorbed by the body's tissues. For the past twenty years, these organ extracts have been derived from the finest organic bovine (cattle), ovine (sheep) and porcine (pig) sources. Different tissue extracts can be combined to achieve different results by targeting specific organs resulting, not only in a revitalizing effect on the target organ per se, but also enhancing the specific function of cellular tissue as well. Practitioners promote for example, thymus gland extract for the immune system, a bovine brain extract for multiple sclerosis, an extract from chicken egg yolks as an anti-infectant, one from frog's eggs for cancer treatment, placenta extracts for women, testicular extracts for men, and the list goes on.

Pharmaceutical companies do have an interest in organ tissues for specific preparations. The classic drug is probably the anti-coagulant Heparin™, used intravenously to prevent blood clotting. It is extracted from the intestinal mucosa of domestic hogs and from the lung tissue of cattle. This is well-characterized biochemically and has an effective antidote. Another interesting analog might be Premarin™ which is an extract from *pregnant mare's urine*, used for hormone replacement in post menopausal women.

This general approach to health and therapeutics has gained more popularity in Europe, even for cancer treatment, but it is more reminiscent of alchemy and witchcraft and leaves much to be desired in the modern age. At best it appears simplistic, more likely a placebo than a panacea, but again it is probably harmless.

Superfoods (Green Foods)

Superfoods are special naturally-occurring foods that contain extraordinary amounts of micro-nutrients, not all of which are yet clearly characterized. They are sometimes called "green foods" and rightfully so, since many superfoods contain extraordinary amounts of the green pigment chlorophyll. But not all superfoods are green foods. Some superfoods have been included on lists of herbs. There is a fine line between "herbs" and "superfoods"; Herbs are medicinal plants that are used primarily in the traditional treatment of sickness and disorders in the body. Many herbs are not encouraged for constant usage, as the body can become tolerant to these healing plants, decreasing their potency when needed. Superfoods on the other hand, are foods that should be regularly supplemented in the diet to complete the body's need for amino acids, trace minerals, vitamins and other nutritional compounds.

Superfoods have been eaten by traditional cultures all over the world from recorded time. Certain cultures have focused on a particular set of superfoods, as they have been readily available in that particular climate. With advancements in modern food technology, it has become possible to carefully dehydrate and store these superfoods for widespread use. That is why many superfoods are not well known, as they have only been available over the past 20 years in different parts of the world.

In traditional societies, superfoods of that culture have been revered foods, taken with ceremony and respect. For example, bee pollen and royal jelly have been traditions of desert cultures, where bee-keeping was common, while in aquatic regions kelps and algaes have been used as dietary supplements, or even mainstays of particular groups. Today's superfoods include grasses, vegetables, whole grains, fruits, herbal extracts and the like. Specific mixtures may be targeted for different conditions but in any case, these superfoods are special in that they provide a natural mix of rich nutrition.

Digestive Aids

The prevalence of gastrointestinal illness is easily illustrated by the fact that in 1998, three of the six most widely prescribed medications in the U.S. were for the treatment of peptic ulcer disease. Common problems from one end of the digestive tract to the other are indeed common. Alternative medicine practitioners have had a field day proposing numerous simplistic theories of how and why these symptoms plague modern society. They have popularized a number of approaches.

Digestive Enzymes. Normal digestion requires specialized protein catalysts we call enzymes to break down the large complex molecules of food into small simple building blocks which are then absorbed in the gut. These digestive enzymes are synthesized and secreted into the gastrointestinal tract, principally from the functioning pancreas. The natural therapists emphasize the importance of food enzymes present especially in uncooked foods, fresh fruits and vegetables, raw sprout grains and even unpasteurized dairy products. They argue that we eat such large quantities of cooked, processed and pasteurized foods that the enzymes our bodies manufacture are too busy digesting *dead* food. As a result, our enzyme reserve can be used up and we then suffer from a host of consequences. The answer for many chronic illnesses is therefore to eat more raw foods and use enzyme supplements.

Trypsin and chymotrypsin are extracted from the pancreas of various animals and then used as a supplement. The enzyme papain (from the papaya fruit) and bromelain (from fresh pineapples) are constantly extracted and used. To protect these preparations from the destructive effect of stomach acid, they are often enteric-coated with something that does not dissolve until it reaches the less acid environment of the intestine. The rationale seems simple enough, but the reality in terms of effectiveness may not be as simple. The gastroenterologists are likely to reserve this approach for exceptional cases.

Friendly Bacteria (Probiotics).   With the widespread use of antibiotics, *Alternative Practitioners* have underscored the potential downside of destroying healthful bacteria in the delicate eco-system of the gut. Again the theory goes, that this unnatural consequence leads to a wide variety of chronic digestive and other metabolic disorders. The answer they have advocated is to use oral supplements of so-called 'friendly bacteria' to restore the necessary ecological balance and promote health.

Oral supplements of *bifido bacterium bifidum*, commonly called bifidus, is used to prevent acute diarrhea in young children, to provide healthful bacteria to human adults, and to re-seed intestinal bacteria affected by diarrhea, chemotherapy, advancing age, antibiotics and other causes. It is the predominant intestinal flora of breast-fed infants. When taken orally, it travels through the colon without multiplication or death, preventing colonization by other organisms. Ingestion of yogurt fermented with bifidus increases the number of bifido bacteria in the stool and suppresses coliform bacteria. Daily consumption of bifidus is usually required to maintain its effectiveness, although effects may persist up to a week or more after its discontinuation. The practice is essentially safe.

Another similar supplement, *lactobacillus acidophilus* is used for improving lactose tolerance as well as for treating vaginal and urinary tract infections, antibiotic-induced diarrhea, oral candida, irritable and inflammatory bowel disorders, and more. Acidophilus (as it is commonly known) is a native inhabitant of the human gastrointestinal tract. It produces lactic acid and hydrogen peroxide, which can suppress disease-causing bacteria. It does not appear to attach to the intestinal tissue. Acidophilus is found in some dairy products, especially milk and yogurt. The practice of supplementation is again essentially safe.

Brewer's Yeast.   Brewer's yeast is obtained as a by-product from the brewing of beer made from an extract of grains and hops. It is included in this section for convenience because it is believed to have some action against *Clostridium difficile* and enterotoxic *E. coli* bacteria, both of which cause diarrhea. It also can reduce the profuse influx of water and electrolyte into the intestine, caused by the *Vibrio cholera* toxin. It is therefore used for the prevention and treatment of acute diarrhea, travelers' diarrhea and diarrhea associated with tube feedings. It has also been commonly used as a source of B vitamins and protein. When used appropriately and for short periods, it is probably quite safe.

HERBAL REMEDIES

Throughout history, people have turned to plants not only for food, shelter and clothing, but also when confronted with disease and pain. Herbal medicine uses the roots, stems, leaves and flowers of plants for medicinal purposes. Over time and through trial and error, herbal medicine expanded into an effective system of health care. Many modern pharmaceutical drugs owe their origins to the discovery of the active ingredients of plants found to have clinical effects. However, with the development of chemically manufactured substances, the use of plant preparations did become somewhat obsolete in this industrial world. Yet, today, as we look for safer healing techniques with fewer side effects and conditions, many are turning back to the natural healing properties of plants.

The herbal dietary supplement market has been growing at an annual rate of 25 percent and is currently estimated at over $5 billion. The market is larger and more mature in Europe, where it is valued in excess of $6 billion. In response to the size and effect of this industry and under mounting pressure from a satisfied public, the government has had to acknowledge the integrity of the emerging herbal therapeutics. A division of the National Institute of Health now has responsibility to promote and fund research into the structure-property relationships and clinical applications for these natural products. Hopefully, there will soon be a separate track for herbal (nutraceutical) preparations to come to the marketplace. This would have to be in contrast to the expensive, new drug application process.

It is also very satisfying to see the new initiatives to improve product consistency of the herbal preparations being dispensed in health food stores and other retail outlets. The new Institute for Nutraceutical Advancement has established the first organized effort to develop and validate analytical testing procedures for botanical raw materials. This is long overdue. Through its Methods Validation Program, several competing companies have come together to fund the needed development of standard QC techniques using the best technical equipment available. Already testing methods have been finalized and are in use for six of the top-selling herbs on the market. Quantitative assays can now determine the concentrations of well-characterized active ingredients. With information like this being made available to the public, the quality of herbal products will only continue to improve and all consumers stand to benefit.

We will now make just a brief introductory review of the more important herbal preparations gaining increasing acceptance in North America.

Ginkgo Biloba

Ginkgo biloba is the oldest living species in the world and ginkgo trees can live as long as one thousand years. Most ginkgo preparations are extracts from the ginkgo leaf. In Chinese medicine, ginkgo is used in the management of various disorders of the central nervous system, as well as respiratory and circulation disorders. In traditional folk medicine, ginkgo has been used as a psychotropic and neurotropic agent. But ginkgo has really made its mark in recent times since credible clinical trials have shown its effect when used orally for stabilization or improvement in brain cognitive function.

It seems that ginkgo extract affects cognitive deficiency in at least two ways: it stimulates the populations of nerve cells that remain functional, and it protects nerve cells from pathologic influences. The identified flavonoid constituents of ginkgo, especially rutin, are known to be free-radical scavengers. Rutin is also known to improve capillary fragility and permeability. Gingko also contains ginkgolide constituents that competitively inhibit platelet-activating factor (PAF) binding at the membrane receptor. This action might be responsible for some reported beneficial effects in asthma, bronchospasm, hypersensitivity reactions, and circulatory diseases.

Ginkgo leaf extract increases cerebral blood flow. That is probably its major appeal since Wellness advocates pontificate on the ability of the body to protect and heal itself. Get blood to flow to the brain and the brain will do the rest. At least, so the theory goes.

The use of ginkgo leaf extract in therapeutic doses might cause mild gastrointestinal complaints, headache, dizziness and allergic skin reactions. Large doses might cause restlessness, diarrhea, nausea, vomiting, lack of muscle tone and weakness. Bleeding is often mentioned as a side effect of ginkgo, but there are very few cases reported.

Ginseng

Ginseng has been used for medicinal purposes for over 2000 years. Approximately 6 million Americans use it regularly. Some people consider the age of the ginseng roots to be important, the older the better. Ginseng is typically used as a tonic to improve well-being and as such, it has been associated with a plethora of physiological benefits. In Chinese medicine it has been used for anemia, diabetes (Type II), gastritis, impotence, fever, etc. In folk medicine, it is used as anti-aging, for gastrointestinal disorders, rheumatism, menopausal symptoms, as an anti-depressant, etc.

The applicable part of ginseng is the root. There are several known active ingredients, the principal class is known as ginsengosides, a number of which are well characterized. Some for example, appear to alter blood pressure as well as lipid, nucleic acid and albumin metabolism. Others stimulate natural killer-cell activity and possibly other immune-system activity, including anti-tumor activity. Some promote growth of normal intestinal flora while inhibiting harmful clostridial species. Many other physiological effects have been noted in over 400 publicized ginseng studies. However, many of these have inadequate study design, or are poorly controlled, or lack standardization. The better studies are indeed suggestive but generally not conclusive.

Echinacea

Echinacea species are native to North America and were used as traditional herbal remedies by the Great Plains Indian tribes. When the settlers came, they too adopted Echinacea for medicinal purposes. In fact, Echinacea was officially listed in the National Formulary from 1916 to 1950. However, with the discovery of antibiotics and the lack of good scientific data to support its use, echinacea fell out of favor. The rising popularity of herbal remedies, the elusive solution to the common cold and the recent advent of antibiotic resistance have all contributed to renewed interest in echinacea.

Principally, echinacea is used today for the symptomatic relief of colds, flu and other upper respiratory infections. It is available in different forms: as a juice, extract, root tincture or tablet. Only recently have reliable quality control methods been used to standardize the preparations. In any case, echinacea is best taken at the earliest signs of developing a cold or flu and then limited to just a few weeks. Contrary to popular belief, there is no evidence for cold proplylaxis if echinacea is used on a continuous basis. That is ill-advised.

Research on the mechanism of action is on-going.

St. John's Wort

St. John's Wort is native to Europe but is commonly found in North America in the dry ground along the roadsides, meadows and woods. The dried, above ground parts have been used in oral preparations for treating depressed mood, anxiety and other secondary symptoms associated with depression such as fatigue, headache, muscle aches, loss of appetite, sleep disturbance etc.

Several active constituents have been isolated from St. John's Wort preparations, all of which may contribute to its pharmacological effects. The precise mechanism of action in depression and the constituents responsible have not been clearly identified. Two constituents that may play a significant role are hypericin and hyperforin. The first of these, hypericin, has been shown to inhibit important enzymes *in vitro*. However, hypericin may not reach adequate concentrations in human tissue to achieve these effects. Hypericin also has affinity for sigma receptors and acts as a receptor antagonist at receptors of the central nervous system. This active ingredient has been identified by the FDA as an investigational new drug and is being studied and developed for the treatment of HIV.

Recently a second constituent hyperforin has been alleged as a probable major player in St. John's Wort's antidepressant activity. It has been shown to modulate the effects of serotonin, possibly through serotonin reuptake inhibition. It is still likely that constituents other than hypericin and hyperforin also contribute to the antidepressant action of St. John's Wort preparations.

Multiple clinical trials have shown that St. John's Wort extracts are superior to placebo, as effective as low dose tricyclic antidepressants, and possibly as effective as fluoxetine (Prozac™) for short-term treatment of mild to moderate major depression. It's probably quite safe when used appropriately.

Kava

Kava (also known as kava, kava) is a herb belonging to the pepper family, and has been used traditionally as a social drink and ceremonial beverage in the South Pacific, somewhat like alcohol is in Western societies. It was reported that even First Lady Hilary Clinton was greeted with quaffs of Kava by the Somoan community during a 1992 Presidential Visit to the island of Oahu. Kava was actually discovered by Captain Cook in the eighteenth century and he named the plant 'intoxicating pepper'.

Kava root extract is now used in the West as a sedative and hypnotic, for the treatment of nervous anxiety, stress and restlessness. The pharmacological activity is believed to result primarily from several arylethylene pyrone constituents (called kava pyrones). Kava's substituted dihydropyrones like methysticin and kavain show evidence of CNS activity but the precise mechanisms of action are not clear. However, a few double-blind clinical trials have demonstrated that kava extracts are superior to placebo and comparable in efficacy to benzodiazepenes for short-term treatment of anxiety disorders and without significant cognitive impairment.

The oral use of kava can cause gastrointestinal complaints, headache, dizziness, enlarged pupils and disturbances of oculomotor equilibrium, and rarely, allergic skin reactions. Chewing kava can cause mouth numbness. Chronic use of 300-400 grams of kava per week can lead to kava dermopathy. This is a pellagra-like syndrome characterized by dry, flaking skin and reddened eyes, as well as temporary yellow discoloration of the skin, hair and nails. The long-term use of large amounts of kava is associated with poor health and should not be advised.

Glucosamine

Glucosamine is not really a herb, but it has found its way into health food stores and drug stores and is used by the same crowd which turns to the herbal remedies. It is actually a glycoprotein derived from marine exoskeletons or produced synthetically. It is required for the synthesis of glycoproteins, glycolipids, and glycosaminoglycans which comprise the body's tendons, ligaments, cartilage, synovial fluid, mucus membranes, and structures in the eye, blood vessels, and heart valves. Glucosamine stimulates metabolism of chondrocyte cells in the articular cartilage and of synoviocytes in the synovial tissues. It has been shown to stop and possibly reverse degenerative joint disease (DJD) although the clinical studies demonstrating its effectiveness have used a patented Italian form of glucosamine sulfate capsules which are not available in the U.S. or Canada. Injected forms of glucosamine are being used in other countries.

Short-term use can cause mild gastrointestinal problems, including nausea, heartburn, diarrhea, constipation, drowsiness, skin reactions, and headache, and the typical dose should not exceed 500mg three times a day. There is concern that glucosamine sulfate products derived from marine exoskeletons might cause reactions in people allergic to shellfish, although no reactions have been reported. Until more is known, people with shellfish allergy should use glucosamine with caution, if at all.

Shark Cartilage

Shark Cartilage is another of those alternative therapies that have become popular due to the widespread exaggerated claims by its proponents and marketers. It is particularly associated with possible reduction in cancer burden. The proponents of shark cartilage as a cancer therapy have claimed that sharks do not get cancer. But they are presumptuous. Researchers report that renal cell carcinoma, lymphoma and cartilage tumors have indeed been identified in sharks. Researchers do theorize however, that shark cartilage might inhibit the process of angiogenesis, preventing the new vessel growth required for solid tumor proliferation. Shark cartilage is known to contain proteins, (40%), glycosaminoglycans (5-20%) and calcium salts, but again its precise mechanisms of action are still unclear.

There is insufficient reliable information available about the safety of shark cartilage. Most shark cartilage on the market is obtained from sharks caught in the Pacific Ocean. Some shark cartilage products have an offensive odor and taste , and can generally cause gastro-intestinal upset. More importantly, however, is the risk of causing or exacerbating hypercalcemia when taken in consistently high risk. That is the principal risk. Phase II clinical trials of shark cartilage for use in prostate cancer and AIDS-related Kaposi's sarcoma reported in 1995 were not completed. Other clinical trials are now underway

The FDA is seeking a permanent injunction against the marketing of one specific brand of shark cartilage. The complaint charges that the product in question is an unapproved drug but is promoted as a treatment for cancer and other diseases. The action against that particular brand of shark cartilage does not affect other brands of shark cartilage that are not intended for use in the treatment of disease and that are otherwise lawfully marketed as mere dietary supplements.

Evening Primrose Oil

Evening Primrose Oil (EPO) is also known as Fever Plant, or Night Willow-Herb. It is used for increasing essential omega-6 fatty acids in the diet, especially gamma linolenic acid. It is obtained from the seed of evening primrose or from borage seeds mainly from Saskatchewan. It is approved in the United Kingdom as a "Prescription Only Medicine" for treating atopic eczema and is approved in Canada as a dietary supplement for increasing essential fatty acid intake. Amongst consumers, there are anecdotal reports of benefits in premenstrual syndrome (PMS) and post-menopause.

It is clear that (EPO) provides significant amounts of gamma linolenic acid (GLA) and linoleic acid. Supplementation with GLA inhibits production of some inflammatory metabolites. It also allows bypassing of the rate-limiting conversion of linoleic acid in food to gamma linolenic acid. Avoiding this step improves the inflammatory/non inflammatory ratio of prostaglandin compounds. Not surprisingly, EPO advocates have therefore promoted its value in immune and auto-immune related conditions. But the hard evidence is still lacking.

EPO is possibly safe when used orally and appropriately. It is usually not toxic even in very large amounts, at least for short periods, but EPO is not advised in pregnancy or nursing, and has also been ill-advised for epileptics.

Garlic

Fresh garlic, garlic powder and garlic oil have been used as flavor components in foods and beverages for a very long time. Traditionally though, garlic has been used as a remedy for colds, flu symptoms and a wide range of conditions. It holds a prominent place in Chinese medicine. It has earned a widespread reputation in the West as something to generally improve health and well-being. Particularly, garlic is now believed to help reduce blood pressure, lower cholesterol, fight infection and somehow enhance the immune system and perhaps even protect against cancer. Some clinical trials with fresh garlic have demonstrated at least marginal benefits.

The applicable parts of garlic are the bulb and clove. Intact garlic cells contain the odorless amino acid, alliin. When intact cells are broken, alliin comes into contact with the enzyme allinase, producing allicin – an unstable, odiferous compound with known antibacterial properties. Further conversion yields some other bioactive principles including ajoene. Aged garlic extract does not contain allicin, but another active component, s-allylcysteine, which prevents experimental physiological aging and age-related immuno-deficiency and atherosclerosis.

Garlic taken orally is generally very safe but it can have dose-related gastrointestinal effects from one end to the other and everything in between. Needless to say, product quality and effectiveness will vary widely due to inconsistencies of raw materials and preparation.

Alfalfa

The ancient Arabs dubbed alfalfa as the "King of the plant

world". It was first used for humans but later became popular with animal feeding. In recent times, its high nutritional value has been rediscovered. The plants have deep roots that penetrate up to forty feet into the soil and the richness derived is harvested essentially in the leaves. As a dietary supplement, the leaves are usually made into a powder after being sun dried, and then a tablet preparation, or else a tea blend or liquid extract, is derived. Young alfalfa sprouts are frequently used in salad preparations.

Traditionally, alfalfa has been used as a diuretic, for urological conditions, for asthma, arthritis and indigestion. It is also a useful source of vitamins A,C,E and K, as well as several minerals and trace minerals. The stems and leaves are presumably safe and specifically, they are reportedly free of some substances found in the alfalfa seeds that are known to trigger lupus (SLE) symptoms.

The dried alfalfa leaves contain about 22% crude fiber. This includes saponins, which appear to help decrease plasma cholesterol without affecting the good HDL levels. The constituents seem to decrease cholesterol absorption and increase excretion of neutral steroids and bileacids. Certain bioflavonoids found in alfalfa may play a role in modulating allergic reactions and the inflammation seen in rheumatoid arthritis. However, the exact mechanism of action is again not now known.

The rich green chlorophyll in the leaves may act as an antioxidant and help to counteract carcinogens. In one review of hundreds of cases of respiratory tract problems, chlorophyll seemed to have a stimulating effect on the lining of the cells, creating a line of defense and also stimulating the granulation tissue for early healing. Alfalfa then may offer an adjunctive treatment to prescription drugs such as antihistamines, bronchodilators and antibiotics. Alfalfa is also a source of beta carotene, the precursor of vitamin A, and has been associated from ancient times with treatment for night blindness.

However, although we know a great deal about the chemical composition of alfalfa, there are still missing variables that render alfalfa something of a nutritional mystery. Its use is probably very safe and in our present junk food culture it is the closest thing to a 'salad in a tablet'.

Valerian

The extracts and essential oil derived from the valerian root are used as flavoring in foods and beverages at levels up to 0.01-0.02%. However, valerian is known to be a sedative and can effectively treat restlessness and sleeping disorders that result from occasional nervous conditions. It is also used for some mood disorders, mild tremors and even attention deficit hyperactivity disorders. It is usually prepared as a steeped tea or as a tincture and used several times a day as necessary for up to several weeks. If valerian is discontinued after prolonged use, it should be tapered to prevent associated withdrawal symptoms.

Valerian can hasten the onset of sleep in individuals who are healthy and individuals with sleep disorders. It can also improve mood and alleviate the difficulty of staying asleep. However, valerian preparations do not seem to produce *immediate* effects like a typical sleep aid. It might take 2 to 4 weeks of use before there is significant improvement, especially in mood. The sedative properties of valerian can be attributed to both the volatile oil and to valepotriate fractions. However, commercial preparations rarely contain valepotriates because valepotriates are heat-sensitive, and chemically unstable. Recent evidence suggested that valerian extract, unlike benzodiazepines, lacked "hangover effects," and did not affect performance, speed or reaction times.

Saw Palmetto

Saw palmetto tea was included in the U.S. pharmacopeia and the National Formulary in the first half of the twentieth century. More importantly, with the increased consciousness and perhaps prevalence of prostate disease in recent time, saw palmetto has emerged as an increasingly popular herbal remedy. Evidence suggests that saw palmetto extract might be useful in Stages I and II of BPH (benign prostatic hyperplasia or hypertrophy). In Stage I of the enlarged prostate, the characteristic symptoms are increased frequency of urination, abnormally frequent urination at night (nocturia), delayed onset of urination and a weak urinary stream. Stage II is characterized by the beginning of decompression of bladder function accompanied by residual urine formation (post-voidal dribbling) and the increased urge to urinate.

BPH can result from increased dihydrotestosterone (DHT) synthesis in the prostate and a shift favoring androgen in the delicate androgen to estrogen ratio. Theoretically, some active ingredient(s) in the saw palemetto can inhibit the binding of DHT at the androgen receptors and/or the activity of the 5-alpha-reductase enzyme on testosterone, which prevents its conversion to DHT in the first place. The use of the saw palmetto berry in patients with BPH can show improvements in symptom scores: frequency, nocturia, residual-urine volumes and measurement of urine flow. But the saw palmetto extract does have **no** significant effect on serum prostate – specific antigen (PSA) levels.

Saw Palmetto is probably safe when used appropriately on a short-term basis. However, prostate problems cannot be taken lightly! Although the link between BPH and prostate cancer is not proven or predictable, all eligible men should have their prostate condition monitored and treated by a qualified medical doctor, wherever indicated or in any doubt whatsoever.

Milk Thistle

There is some irony in the convenient name of this final herbal remedy in the context of this book. Milk thistle is neither a dairy product nor a derivative of anything dairy. It gets its name in part from the milky sap which exudes from the broken leaves of the milk thistle plant. The plant was once grown in Europe as a vegetable for salads and as a substitute for spinach. Actually, the supplement is derived from the fruit or seed.

The most common milk thistle product, known as Silymarin, is a complex extract from the fruit and seed. It consists of four favanolignans which are known to exhibit liver protective and antioxidant effects. It is believed that the therapeutic activity of silymarin is based on at least two mechanisms of action. The first of these involves an alteration of the outer liver cell membrane that prevents toxin penetration. The second involves the stimulation of the nucleolar polymerase A, resulting in increased ribosomal protein synthesis. This can in principle, stimulate the formation of new liver cells. Therefore milk thistle extract has been used most often as some kind of remedy for gastrointestnal illness and especially for liver disease. Some clinical studies support the claim of benefits for those with different kinds of liver condition.

Milk thistle is probably quite safe when used appropriately.

That's enough about milk thistle and about all these so-called natural products, complementary therapies and alternative healing professions.

Could it be that we have yet to explore a real goldmine of nature that has until very recently, eluded those in search of natural solutions to enhance good health and even deal with different chronic conditions? Perhaps it's because the therapeutic treasures are hidden beneath the surface of nature awaiting good scientific investigation.

So the question before the house comes down to the simple probing inquiry:

"WHATEVER BECAME OF MILK?"

Chapter Two

THE MILK CONTROVERSY
Panacea or Poison?

Yes, whatever became of Milk?

The huge dairy industry in the West is alive and well. But it is engaged in a heated war of words, science and economics. On one side there are powerful, vocal industry advocates and their lobby defending "the perfect food" that "has something for everybody". On the other, passionate opponents of the dairy establishment may not be as organized but they are taking their cause directly to the public. They are enlisting an increasing number of professionals who now question the real nutritional value of milk and even go further to attribute negative health consequences to its human consumption. For some then, it's almost a nutritional panacea while for others, it is not very short of being a dietary poison.

THE STORY OF MILK

Milk in Society
What is unambiguous, is the absolute value of the fluid secreted from the mammary glands of female mammals for their *immediate offspring*. It is the ideal nourishment, designed and produced by nature for those particular young ones, for the period beginning right after birth. But the milk of domesticated animals has become an important food source for *humans*, either as a fresh fluid or processed into a variety of dairy products such as butter and cheese.

Almost all the milk now consumed in the Western hemisphere is from the *cow*, and milk and dairy products have become very important commercial items. Other important sources of milk are *the sheep and goat*, which are especially important in Southern Europe and the Mediterranean area; *the water buffalo*, which is widely domesticated in Asia; and *the camel*, which is important in the Middle East and North America. Milk and Dairy products are promoted in the West by dieticians and nutritionists (as well as by Dairy Marketing Boards) as one of the four major Food Groups necessary for adequate nutrition. The other Food Groups are (i) Cereals and Grains, (ii) Fruits and Vegetables, and (iii) Meat, Poultry and Fish. (It's about time that we recognized a 'Fifth Food Group' in modern society: Fast, Convenience and Junk Foods, prepared for the consumer's pleasure and that industry's profit.) It is clear that orthodoxy has placed dairy products in the core of human nutrition, at least for people living on this side of the world. However, it may be surprising to learn that most of the human beings that live on planet Earth do not drink or use cow's milk. Many cannot do so comfortably, even if they wished, because of lactose intolerance, food allergies and other conditions which could make them ill.

But North America is a continent of milk drinkers. In this society, one of the most sacred of all 'sacred cows' is the *milk* of the cow itself. It's more American than apple pie and as Canadian as pure maple syrup. Even in Mexico, it has established its place and is remarkably more popular than the famous tequila. Everything to do with dairy food and especially that of milk, is surrounded with emotional and cultural importance.

For each of us, milk was indeed our very first food. If we were fortunate, it was our mother's milk for the first few months of life, and up to one year in some cases. This is nature's special link, given and taken with love, bonding each generation to the next! Here in the West, if it was not mother's milk, it was some form of cow's milk or soy milk "formula". Milk was the only path to survival. And then, as little infants are weaned, most parents would not conceive of raising their children without the perceived benefit of cow's milk to help their little bones and their fragile bodies to grow big and strong. It all seems so natural. The pure white, silky texture (so exploited by advertising) is the epitome of society's concept of wholesome purity and good health.

Classical nutrition education in our schools and massive advertising in the media then reinforce the central nutritional role for milk. The repeated health emphasis in the ever present advertising gives many the impression that such commercials are mere public service announcements and not sales and marketing initiatives. Cow's milk is made to seem just so normal. Who would deny the self-evident assertions of dairy advertising. "Milk is good for your body." "It's the perfect food". "It's an essential food group". "You've got to have milk, where else will you get your calcium?" "Drink a glass of milk a day". "Drink at least three glasses of milk each day". "Oh, there's nothing like a warm glass of milk". Just the thought of milk in our culture connotes health and satisfaction to so many consumers. The message is so effective that one in every seven dollars spent in the grocery goes to buy dairy products. With the typical North American consuming almost 400lbs (180 kg) pounds of dairy products each year, this industry means billions and billions of dollars annually. It is supported and promoted by massive advertising, political lobbying, nutritional education and a huge public relations effort. All this has created the widely-held perception and indeed conviction that **milk** is the real nutritious thing!

Speaking of the real…thing, soft drink manufacturers have gone head-to-head in competitive advertising for market share. Carbonated soft drinks – average consumption of which is now more than double what it was in 1970 – are likely displacing beverage milks in the diet. Especially so, as more and more meals are eaten away from home – increasing the appeal of fast, convenience and junk foods, including soft drinks. At the same time, consumers' preference for carbonated beverages and the concern about extra calories and dietary fat by many women, are important factors in the decreased consumption of fluid milk since the 1970's.

According to U.S. food intake survey data, the intake of both regular and low-calorie soft drinks has increased dramatically since the 1970's. That increase is highest among teenagers and young adults, with women drinking more low-calorie drinks. Annual food supply data show that per capita consumption of regular carbonated soft drinks *increased* from 22 gallons in 1970, to 40 gallons in 1994 and to 41 gallons in 1997; while that from diet drinks increased from 2 gallons in 1970 to 12 gallons in 1994 and 1997. By comparison, annual per capita consumption of beverage milks *declined* from 31 gallons in 1970 to 25 gallons in 1994 and 24 gallons in 1997.

Or consider this: in 1945, Americans drank more than four times as much milk as compared to carbonated soft drinks; but in 1997, they downed nearly two and a half times more soda than milk. On any given day, half of all Americans drank carbonated soft drinks in 1994-96. You can now see who has won that advertising war.

To help consumers include more dairy products in the diet, a number of promotional campaigns have been developed by the Federal Government, by private and public dairy interests, and by health professionals concerned about the impact on nutritional health. Some of these activities target specific groups of North Americans to improve intake of dairy products overall; others are more focused on the nutrient contributions (especially calcium) and the link to health. Just think of the celebrity endorsements, of 'the milk mustache', or the cow billboards, or slogans like "milk makes sense" because "milk has something for everyone" However, the basic goal of each campaign is to promote more and more dairy product consumption. That may be today a confluence of interests in the industry's wealth as much as in the nation's health.

But let's go back to the beginning.

Milk In History

The story of milk began thousands of years ago with the oldest known civilizations. Historians and archaeologists tell us that man probably began domesticating animals between 8000 and 5000 B.C. They believe that cattle were first used as sources of food in Asia or northeast Africa. The dairy cow, as we know her today, is a descendent of those ancient cattle.

The earliest record suggesting man's use of milk from animals as food was unearthed in a temple in the Euphrates Valley near Babylon. There an archaeologist found a mosaic frieze believed to be about 5,000 years old. It showed a shelter built of reeds; men milking cows; and milk being poured through a crude strainer into stone jars.

Milk and foods made from milk are mentioned in the Bible (speaking of a land, flowing with *milk* and honey. By the way, someone has pointed out that milk and honey are the only two substances on earth with the sole purpose of being a food). Early Hindu writings and hymns often refer to milk and foods made from it. Ancient Greeks, Romans and Egyptians recorded their use of milk in religious ceremonies, and as a medicine. The Vikings carried large supplies of butter on their sea voyages. In the thirteenth century, Marco Polo wrote that the strong Tartar armies enjoyed a fermented form of mare's milk. Christopher Columbus described his landing in the New World in1492, 'It was wonderful to see…land for cattle, although they have none.'

The story of milk in North America is summarized in Table 1.

Table 1.   The Milk Story in North America

1518	First domestic cattle arrive in New World but none survive.
1608	Cows reach Plymouth Colony at Cap Tourmente
1660	Cows arrive in New France from Brittany and Normandy
1834	Anglo-American inventor Jacob Perkins obtains a British patent for the first refrigerator unit.
1856	Gail Borden received first patent on condensed milk from the United States and England.
1890	Test for fat content of milk and cream perfected by Dr. S.M. Babcock.
1908	First compulsory pasteurization law (Chicago) applying to all milk except that from tuberculin-tested cows.
1919	Homogenized milk premieres successfully on East Coast.
1932	Way of increasing vitamin D in milk made practical.
1932	First plastic-coated paper milk cartons introduced commercially.
1942	Home milk delivery begins (initially as a war conservation measure).
1948	Ultra-high temperature pasteurization is introduced.
1964	Plastic milk container introduced commercially.
1973	Only 10% of Americans still receive home milk delivery. By 1995, fewer than one percent of American homes are visited by the milkman.
1974	Nutrition labeling of fluid milk products.
1980	American Dairy Association launches the national introduction of the "REAL" (R) Seal dairy symbol.
1985	Program picturing lost children on milk cartons begins January 1. Within a month, more than 400 dairies nationwide are participating. Lower-fat dairy products gain widespread acceptance.
1994	Nutrition Labeling and Education Act requires mandatory nutrition labeling.
1994	National Fluid Milk Processor Promotion Board launches "Milk, What a Surprise!" campaign. The latest trend–everyone's wearing a milk mustache.

1995	Milk consumption among Americans *rises* for the first time in 25 years.
1996	Its second year, the National Fluid Milk Processor Promotion Board relaunches its national, education initiative with a new tagline "Milk, Where's *Your* Mustache?" New celebrities and programs are introduced targeting men, college-age students and teens.

It is a story dictated as much by the advertising and promotion programs in the marketplace, as by the changing technology in the field. In four hundred years, cow's milk has remained cow's milk, and we have only learned to preserve it, process it and promote it. It is still a product of nature. The first domestic cattle were brought to the New World in 1518 and landed at Sable Island, but none survived. Samuel de Champlain brought the first cattle which survived in the early seventeenth century. A farm was established for his colony at Cap Tourmente in New England. The farm still exists but it is no longer a dairy farm. In 1660, good breeding cows arrived in New France from Brittany and Normandy. These became the foundation stock for the only breed of dairy cattle developed in Canada...the Canadienne. Some Quebec farms are still stocked with herds bred from descendants of those sturdy, productive animals.

Today, after careful selective breeding and genetic screening, North American purebred cattle are internationally renowned. Many are exported to start or improve herds in other parts of the world. Of all the registered purebreds, the Holstein-Freisian which originated in the provine of Friesland in the Netherlands, now make up the overwhelming majority. They are the largest cows of all breeds, averaging about 1430lbs (650kg) and are easily distinguished black and white cows, with distinct markings. They produce on average about ten times their weight (as much as 14,000lbs, 6300kg) of milk on an annual basis. They are hardy animals which acclimatize well and produce consistent, superior milk.

From farm to processing plant, modern dairying is an important North American industry. Both the U.S. and Canada rank in the top ten in total milk production among the major milk producing countries. Many years of superior breeding, improved feeding, and efficient farming methods have increased the quantity, and improved the qualityof of milk supplied by North American cows.

Millions of North Americans now depend on the dairy industry for all, or part of their livelihood. About one billion hectolitres of milk are produced by about thirty million dairy cows on half a million farms across North America. This milk is processed and packaged in thousands of plants and sold as a variety of fluid milks and an even wider variety of dairy products.

Dairy plants process about 35% of the milk supply as fluid milk and cream; about 30% as creamery butter (and skim milk powder, a by-product of butter production); about 28% as cheese; and about 7% as ice cream mix and concentrated milks. A considerable amount of skim milk powder and evaporated milk is exported from the U.S. and Canada each year, as vital parts for example, of Food Aid programs to the developing world.

The Dairy Cow

The dairy cow is the most valuable milk producing animal and is central to the entire dairy industry. It provides about ninety percent of the world's milk supply. No other animal yields as much as the dairy cow, which is the main source of milk supply in North America where so much of the pasture, climate and terrain are very suitable. And why do we get our milk for human consumption from the cow? Perhaps only because of the coincidence of three factors: its docile nature, its huge size and its abundant milk supply. The choice seems so appropriately blessed by nature and our culture. We are conditioned to think and feel this way.

The amount of milk a cow produces depends on her diet, breed, age and stage of lactation. Cows are milked twice daily for 305 days of the year. A good 'milker' will give about 7 gallons (27 litres) each day. For the remaining 60 days, the cow is dry and not milked. This period gives her time to rest and store important body-building nutrients before her calf is born. She gives birth to a calf yearly. Crudely stated, **the diary cow is essentially a milk production machine in the service of man.** If in India she is sacred, in the West she is exploited and hopefully in other places, she is simply respected as an animal. But then, considered another way, that may be her 'raison d'être' – her divinely appointed mission. Does the cow find her own measure of 'self-actualization' in the process of perpetual milk production? And then again, she does not even have the comfort and satisfaction of her young calf at her breast, but must contend with the cold, artificial, mechanical milking devices almost all the time. Yet, she is making a difference – a big difference, as we shall now see.

MILK IN THE LIFE CYCLE

A cow's milk is obviously designed for that young calf which she gives birth to each year. It is her baby's milk. Breast-feeding is the natural way for all mammals. Part of the very definition of a mammal is that the female of the species has milk-producing glands in her breasts which provide nourishment for her offspring. Each species produces a unique mammary gland secretion designed specifically to strengthen the immune system and provide nourishment for her own kind. Mammalian babies are weaned naturally after their birth weight has approximately tripled. By then, nature apparently has run its course. But animals in the service of humans are utilized to feed large populations, even in the development of 'infant formula' to substitute for human breast milk.

Infant formulas are generally based on some type of cow's milk, modified with water and sugar to make the protein and carbohydrate content more similar to human milk. Commercial formulae made from cow's milk contain insufficient amounts of iron and vitamin C and obviously lack some of the trace nutritional ingredients unique to human milk. For newborns and infants, formulae are a distant second and an inadequate alternative to the ideal – human breast milk!

Breast Feeding

The American Academy of Pediatrics and the Canadian Pediatric Society have been staunch advocates of human breast feeding as the optimal nutrition for infants. It is the foundation of all good feeding practices. Extensive research has documented diverse and compelling advantages to infants, mothers, families and society at large from breast feeding and the use of *human* milk for infant feeding. These include health, nutritional, immunologic, developmental, psychological, social, economic and even environmental benefits.

Human milk is uniquely superior for infant feeding and is species-specific; all substitute feeding options differ markedly from it. The research shows that human milk and breast feeding of infants provide advantages with regard to general health, growth and development, while significantly decreasing the risks for a large number of acute and chronic diseases.

Despite the demonstrated benefits of breastfeeding, there are some exceptional situations in which breastfeeding is not in the best interest of the infant. These include the infant with galactosemia, the infant whose mother uses illegal drugs, or has untreated active tuberculosis, or who (in North America) has been infected with HIV.

Increasing the rates of breastfeeding (initiation and duration) is a national health objective. The target has recently been to 'increase to at least 75% the proportion of mothers who breastfeed their babies in the early post-partum period, and to at least 50% the proportion who continue breastfeeding until their babies are 5 to 6 months old.' The percentage of women in the U.S. who were breastfeeding, either exclusively or in combination with formula feeding, at the time of hospital discharge was below 60% as recently as 1995.

The pediatricians have made clear recommendations about breastfeeding practices that deserve to be promoted everywhere. Human milk is the preferred feeding for all infants, including premature and sick newborns, with only rare exceptions. It should begin as early as possible after birth, usually within the first hour. Nursing should be on demand, at signs of hunger, and no supplements should be given unless medically indicated. Newborns should be seen by a doctor or their appointee at 2-4 days, for reassessment and reconfirmation of good breastfeeding practice. Infants weaned before 12 months of age should **not** receive cow's milk feedings but should receive iron-fortified infant formula. Vitamin D and iron may need to be given before 6 months of age in selected infants. Should hospitalization of the breastfeeding mother or infant be necessary, every effort should be made to maintain breastfeeding by one means or another.

Colostrum

Some *natural* health promoters have recently been trying to market colostrum from cows as an 'immune-boosting, life enhancing, healing agent' for human adults. Colostrum is the pre-milk fluid produced from the mammary glands during the first 24-48 hours after birth. But it is obviously nature's 'warm-up act' – produced for a defined population, for a defined period, with a defined purpose. To extend that population, or period, or purpose requires adequate scientific justification which to this author's opinion has not been forthcoming. It is a long step (and perhaps a leap of faith) to extrapolate analytical results from the chemistry of fresh colostrum, to physiological effects of commercial products months and years later in the general population.

Yet promoters of colostrum would like the public to believe that colostrum as a food supplement would help rebuild the immune system; destroy viruses, bacteria and fungi; accelerate healing of all body tissue; lose weight by burning fat; increase bone and lean muscle mass; slow down and even reverse aging! Only good *science* can make that case. The issues of human need, sourcing, supply, quality control, stability, active ingredients and their concentrations, biological availability, biochemical and physiological mechanisms of action, safety, standardization and more, have not been adequately addressed.

The unwarranted claims derived (by association and extrapolation) from limited research data does no scientific justice to the known facts. They cannot justify widespread use of any colostrum food supplement as a responsible health practice. Colostrum may be 'life's first food' as some promoters are eager to point out, but it is neither life's only food, life's adult food or life's best food. It remains nature's 'warm-up act' for newborn babies…and only that!

Children

The transition form breastfeeding or formula to fluid milk and solid foods is a gradual process that most infants accomplish sometime between 6 and 12 months of age. During the preschool years, the soft, bland diet of infancy gradually undergoes change. The preschool child learns to eat foods with a variety of flavors and textures, and begins to establish food habits which may permanently influence future nutritional status. In the second year of life, a child's rate of growth slows and appetite usually decreases. Although energy needs in relation to body weight are lower than in infancy, a continuing supply of high quality protein and other growth-promoting nutrients are required. Throughout preschool years, although the child's bones and teeth will develop at a slower rate than earlier, substantial amounts of calcium, phosphorous and vitamin D are still needed. Most dieticians would agree that milk plays an important role in supplying these nutrients, even though a child's decreased appetite may mean that he or she is drinking much less than the daily 2 to 3 servings recommended. Food made with milk and commercial dairy products such as yogurt, cheese and ice cream can be introduced in the preschool years.

The school age child's rapid rate of growth, with a corresponding increase in their appetite, demands even more food to meet their body's needs. Again, dairy foods are considered to make a significant contribution in terms of calcium, riboflavin and high quality protein, plus other nutrients.

Adolescents and Teens

A youngster's rapid growth and development during prepubertal and pubertal years brings about a marked increase in all their nutrient needs. Requirements for energy, vitamins and high quality protein are greater, and the needs for calcium and iron are at a higher level than at any other period of life, except perhaps during pregnancy and lactation. When this age group includes a few servings of milk and milk products in their daily diet, they obtain generous amounts of many essential nutrients, particularly calcium, riboflavin, niacin and protein. The vitamin D needed by these growing young people is also provided from the recommended intake of fortified milk.

Some adolescents, whose eating habits were good in earlier childhood, succumb to fad diets and unusual food practices during their teen years. Changes in food patterns may reflect a desire to assert independence and to exert authority in food selections. They try to copy a peer group, or to achieve certain goals related to their figure, skin, general fitness and appearance. Whatever their meal patterns, all teenagers should be encouraged to include at least a wide variety of foods each day. Those who are calorie conscious should be advised to select all

foods with care to ensure an adequate supply of all the essential nutrients. Skim and partly skimmed (2%) milk, with their high ratio of nutrients to total calories, are then a better choice than regular homogenized
milk.

The teenage girl should take special care to cultivate good food
habits in order to build a healthy body so that she may possibly bear
healthy babies later. At the same time, she should gain the essential
knowledge needed to select proper foods for her future family. Most
teenage boys have better appetites than teenage girls; as a result, they
are more likely to eat larger and more nutritious meals. In addition to
their greater body size, boys tend to be more active, and often take part
in more strenuous athletic activities than girls. Thus, their energy needs
are higher and their energy requirements greater. The need for most
essential nutrients for both boys and girls does not decrease until they
stop growing during their late teens or early twenties. In young adult-
hood, their food choices are still most important. Dieticians often suggest that milk and milk products will serve both teenage girls and boys
well, and provide an easy solution to many of their nutrient needs.

Adults

Adults require the same nutrients as children or adolescents,
but in different proportions. Their needs are essentially for maintenance of health and vigor, rather than for growth and development.
Energy requirements are usually less, depending upon one's daily work
and activity. At any age, the body must have in particular, a constant
supply of calcium. When adequate sources of calcium are not included
in the diet, during the later adult years, the body may have to deplete the
bones (the calcium "bank") to obtain the needed amounts of this essential nutrient. Recent studies suggest that even moderate calcium deficiencies over a prolonged period may lead to bone fragility (osteoporosis) in later years. Therefore, the knee jerk response given by authorities is to drink more milk or use other dairy products to protect those
bones. We will return to this important but somewhat controversial
question in Chapter Ten.

The average adult can, in principle at least, obtain the necessary calcium intake by including the recommended 2 or 3 servings of

milk and milk products in the daily diet. These foods will also provide generous amounts of other important essentials for the healthy, active adult. Skim or partly skimmed milks are the better food choices for weight watchers.

Mothers

The expectant mother should be guided from the early stages in her selection of foods by a physician who is aware of her general health and the progress of her pregnancy. Studies indicate that the food she eats affects the course of pregnancy, the health of the newborn infant, and the mother's ability to nurse her baby. The teenage mother must give particular consideration to her daily meals, since the extra requirements of pregnancy are superimposed on her own nutritional needs as she completes normal growth and reaches maturity.

In human development, the most rapid rate of growth occurs in the unborn infant. An increased supply of several nutrients is required after the first three months, both for the developing fetus, and to build up the mother's reserves in preparation for childbirth and lactation. If the mother has been well nourished before her pregnancy, the increased recommended allowances will be adequate to protect her health and that of her unborn baby. Otherwise, dietary improvements should begin as soon as she is aware of her condition.

Calcium and phosphorous are needed for the formation of bone and tooth structures throughout pregnancy. Although most of the deposition of these minerals in both bones and teeth takes place during the last trimester of pregnancy, the infant's first (baby) teeth begin to form early in prenatal life. To meet these extra requirements, additional calcium is recommended during the second and third trimesters, even though absorption of dietary calcium improves during pregnancy. Increased milk and milk products are recommended by dieticians at this time to contribute the additional calcium and phosphorus needed, and simultaneously to provide extra protein needed for development of the fetus, and for formation of new maternal tissues. The vitamin D required to ensure proper utilization of the minerals can be obtained from fortified milk or from a vitamin supplement prescribed by the physician.

Dairy foods continue to play an important role in the mother's meal pattern after her baby is born, particularly while she is nursing the child. Although lactating women are usually advised to include about the same amount of dairy foods in their daily meals as pregnant women (3-4 servings), the new mother's needs for some nutrients are increased during the lactation period. Extra protein, B vitamins, and vitamins A and C are particularly important, while her requirements for calcium, iron and vitamin D are the same as during pregnancy.

Seniors

Senior citizens must continue their respect for good nutrition if they wish to enjoy good health in their later years. Fundamentally, the older adult's nutrient needs are very similar to those of younger persons. Less physical activity usually results in decreased energy needs to avoid obesity and its complications. Decreased appetite, inadequate mastication of food, less efficient digestion, poor absorption and utilization of nutrients, may also accompany the aging process. Again, dieticians would point out that the excellent nutrient content of dairy foods, with comparatively moderate energy value, makes them important food choices for this age group. Older persons who do not enjoy drinking milk can benefit from its food values by using it in food preparation, or by eating cheese, ice cream, yogurt and other dairy foods. These are sources of more easily-digested, high quality protein and fat, plus a variety of other essentials, including the calcium needed to protect against any further demineralization of the skeleton, which too often results in osteoporosis.

MILK AND TECHNOLOGY

Modern technology has made it possible for the dairy industry to offer a wide variety of milk products to North Americans. Research into these products continues in an effort to satisfy the preferences of consumers; to find effective use of surpluses and by-products; to facilitate better storage, distribution and marketing methods; and to maintain even higher standards of quality.

Pasteurization

Pasteurization is a heat treatment process devised by the French chemist Louis Pasteur around 1865 to inhibit the natural fermentation of milk and wine. Pasteurization is one of the most important steps in processing milk. It greatly improves milk's "keeping" quality by effectively destroying virtually all the disease-producing (and most other) bacteria. The harmless lactic acid bacteria that cause milk to go sour, survive pasteurization but can be destroyed when milk is heated to ultra high temperatures (135 to 140°C). Milk to be used for fluid purposes or in the manufacture of most dairy foods is pasteurized. There is still a small demand for raw milk cheddar cheese; however, bacteria are destroyed during the cheese manufacturing process. Normally, pasteurization does not affect the quality or the quantity of calcium, protein, riboflavin and vitamin A present in fluid milk, but some vitamin C and thiamin are destroyed at the high pasteurization temperatures.

Fluid milk is usually pasteurized by one of two methods. The most modern, used by the majority of dairies, is known as "High Temperatures, Short Time" (HTST) pasteurization. Milk is heated to not less than 72°C and held for not less than 16 seconds; then it is cooled rapidly to 4.44°C. For maximum flavor retention, large dairies report that pasteurization temperatures do not exceed 79.4°C. The other method, used in small plant operations, involves heating the milk to at least 62.7°C holding it for not less than 30 minutes, then cooling it rapidly to 4.44°C. Milk, should then be stored below 10°C. Pasteurized milk that is kept refrigerated in closed containers will remain consumable for approximately 14 days.

A very special way to pasteurize milk is called UHT (Ultra High Temperature). In this process, the milk is heated to at least 138°C for not less than 2 seconds. Then it is cooled quickly down to 2°C. This milk is almost sterilized: there are virtually no bacteria left. The milk is packaged usually in rectangular boxes under aseptic conditions. It can then be stored unopened, at room temperature for up to six months. Once opened it needs to be kept in the refrigerator and will again last for about 14 days.

Raw milk is not recommended. However, in homes or communities where raw milk is available, health authorities strongly advise home pasteurization. Milk should be heated to the verge of

boiling, then cooled rapidly.

Homogenization

Raw milk is an oil-in-water *emulsion*, with the fat globules dispersed in a continuous skim milk phase. The mixture is stabilized by complex phospholipids and proteins bound to the surface of the fat globules. If this raw milk were left to stand, however, the fat would rise and form a cream layer. Homogenization is a mechanical treatment of the fat globules in milk brought about by passing milk under high pressure through a tiny orifice, which results in a decrease in the average diameter and an increase in number and surface area, of the fat globules. The net result, from a practical point of view, is a much reduced tendency for creaming of fat globules. Three factors contribute to this enhanced stability of homogenized milk: a decrease in the mean diameter of the fat globules (a factor in Stokes Law); a decrease in the size distribution of the fat globules (causing the speed of rise to be similar for the majority of globules, such that they don't tend to cluster during creaming); and an increase in density of the globules (bringing them closer to the continuous phase) due to the adsorption of a protein membrane. In addition, heat pasteurization breaks down the cryo-globulin complex, which tends to cluster fat globules causing them to rise.

It is most likely that a combination of two different theories explains the reduction in size of the fat globules during the homogenization process. The first is called turbulence. Energy, dissipating in the liquid milk going through the homogenizer valve, generates intense turbulent circulatory forces (called eddy currents) of the same size as the average globule in diameter. Globules are thus torn apart by these Eddy currents thereby reducing their average size. The second theory of cavitation emphasizes the considerable pressure drop with the change of velocity of fluid. The liquid milk cavitates because its vapor pressure is attained and cavitation generates further eddies that would produce disruption of the fat globules. Both effects take place simultaneously. In any case, the high velocity gives the milk a high kinetic energy which is disrupted in a very short period of time. Increased pressure increases velocity. Dissipation of this energy leads to a high energy density (energy per volume and time). The resulting small diameter of the fat globules is a function of that energy density.

More important to health perhaps, is what happens on the surface of these tiny fat globules. The milk fat globule has a native membrane, picked up at the time of secretion, made of amphiphilic molecules with both hydrophilic and hydrophobic sections. This membrane lowers the interfacial tension resulting in a more stable emulsion. During homogenization, there is a tremendous increase in surface area and the native milk fat globule membrane (MFGM) is lost. However, there are many amphiphilic molecules present from the milk plasma that readily adsorb. These include casein micelles (partly spread) and whey proteins. Also found in this new surface layer is an enzyme called xanthine oxidase (XO) which is designed to aid fat digestion in the gut of the baby calf. When milk is homogenized for human consumption, this enzyme accompanies the absorption of the tiny fat globules through the human intestinal wall. When it gets into the human circulation, it has been shown to damage the blood vessel walls and helps initiate the early stages of atherosclerosis. The consequences can be serious. Cardiologist Kurt Oster studied 75 patients with angina in the early 1970's. When all the patients were taken off milk and given folic acid and vitamin C to combat the action of xanthine oxidase, the results were dramatic. Chest pains decreased and symptoms lessened. Dr. Kurt Esselbacher, a prominent Harvard cardiologist has observed that "homogenized milk, because of its XO content, is one of the major causes of heart disease in the U.S." This is not an extreme view by any means. A pathologist has reviewed the coronary vessels of over 1500 children and adolescents who had died as a result of accidents, and found many of them had signs of early atherosoleroisis. More particularly, the majority of children with normal coronaries had been breast-fed, whereas the majority of children with the diseased vessels had been fed cow's milk or cow's milk-based formula. The association was not remote.

Homogenization of whole milk then may be a double-edged innovation. It is essential to the dairy industry if milk is to be marketed as a fluid on a regular basis in modern urbanized communities. This way the milk can be kept fresh and not sour easily. But it may be at a small price – or at a big one – if xanthine oxidase thus becomes a disguised silent killer for some consumers predisposed to atheroseloerosis and then heart disease or stroke.

Derivatives

Cow's Milk has given rise to a long line of dairy products that now includes many variations of fluid milks, milk powders, butter, cheese, creams (including popular ice cream), and yogurt. This diversity has sustained and expanded the dairy industry and thanks to good technology, has enhanced the public perception of dairy as a safe, high quality, nutritious component of the family diet. There's something for everybody.

The impact of technology on the milk supply has also permitted the isolation of different commercial ingredients with unique characteristics and applications. Table 2 is an abbreviated summary of some of these milk/whey ingredients and their potential usefulness on the market. These are made possible through the application of advanced techniques like coagulation and precipitation, microfiltration, chromatography, reverse osmosis and others. The ingredients listed include different types of protein isolates, enzymes, immunoglobulins, minerals and lactose. And that list is by no means exhaustive. Each product is fully characterized and with quality specifications. They find different applications in industry mainly as recipe ingredients in all kinds of food products as well as in consumer use as food supplements. The dairy industry is consistently supporting and partially funding more research in pursuit of new developments to exploit the rich value of milk – the goldmine of nature.

MILK NUTRIENTS

Milk is a complex mixture. It contains proteins in colloidal dispersion, lactose in true solution, minerals, fat-soluble and water-soluble vitamins, enzymes and other organic compounds. This makes milk a truly unique liquid food. Its white appearance is produced by two salts, calcium caseinate and calcium phosphate. All dairy foods are derived from milk, and their essential components are the same as those of milk but in varying amounts. Butter is an exception being comprised mainly of milk fat.

By very efficient marketing methods, the dairy industry has established milk and milk products as an essential part of any complete

TABLE 2. COMMERCIAL MILK/WHEY INGREDIENTS

Whey Protein Isolates
For nutritional applications requiring excellent amino acid profiles, high solubility, free from flavor, fat and lactose.   Available in spray dried and instant forms.

Whey Protein Concentrate
High nutritional value, excellent flavor and solubility. Strong water retention and good emulsification properties.

Specialty Whey Proteins
A unique whey protein designed with enhanced heat stability, gelation, and water binding properties. Excellent flavor and solubility.

Rennet Casein
Natural milk protein, excellent oil binding and structure forming properties.

Acid Casein
The ideal milk protein for applications in emulsified products.

Milk Protein Concentrates
Natural milk protein, excellent replacement for non-fat milk powder.

Lactoferrin
Biologically active protein for immune stimulation, iron supplementation, probiotic activity and antibacterial applications.

Lactoperoxidase
Natural food system preservations, natural antimicrobial activity for use in specialized applications.

Immunoglobulins
A purified, highly active isolate of *bovine immunoglobulins* with immune enhancing and antibody binding activity for cow's antigens.

Milk Minerals
Natural source of milk calcium also containing high levels of other minerals.

Lactose
Milk sugar with low sweetness and an excellent flavor profile with improved browning and yield improvement.

and balanced diet in the Western world. It is labeled as such, specifically designated as you know, to be one of the four essential Food Groups. This is a mere formal classification, not universally accepted by any means. But it is central to nutrition education in the home, the school, the media and the society as a whole.

What are the nutritional ingredients of milk? What justifies its reputation as 'the perfect food' with 'something for everyone'?

Proteins

Bovine milk's principal proteins are casein (about 80%) and the whey proteins called alpha-lactalbumin, beta-lactoglobulin, serum albumen and lactoferrin. These proteins are complete or high quality; that is, they contain in good proportions all the essential amino acids required by man. Essential amino acids are those that must be provided in food because the body cannot synthesize them to the degree sufficient to meet the needs for growth and maintenance. There is even a protein quality scale based on casein as standard: the casein equivalent ration (CER). Most other animal proteins are also complete, whereas plant proteins are often incomplete and have a lower biological value. Soy protein, for example, which is probably the best plant protein source, is low in one essential amino acid called methionine.

Cheese is also an excellent source of high quality protein, derived essentially from casein. But since it does not contain whey proteins, its amino acid contribution differs from that of milk. Milk protein has a high coefficient of digestibility (87 to 90%). In addition, when combinations of foods are eaten at the same meal, milk's high quality protein complements the incomplete proteins. For example, milk contains lysine to supplement the amino acids in bread. Together these foods can present more amino acids in ideal proportions for protein synthesis in the body than either food by itself.

But it has often been pointed out that we tend to ingest too much protein (albeit the wrong type and sources of protein) on a daily basis in North America. This has important consequences for health and we will therefore return to this question as it pertains to the pros and cons of consuming milk and dairy products, later in this chapter.

Fats (Lipids)

Milk fat is 95 to 96% triglycerides (esters of fatty acids with glycerol); 0.8 to 1.0% phospholipids; 0.2 to 0.4% sterol – chiefly cholesterol; traces of free fatty acids, waxes and squalene (an intermediary of cholesterol); and varying amounts of all the known fat-soluble vitamins. The complex composition of milk fat includes at least 64 different fatty acids, containing from 4 to 26 carbon atoms with a relatively high proportion of short-chain, saturated fatty acids, many of which are not found in other fats.

In general, the fatty acids in milk fat are about 66% saturated, 30% monounsaturated and 4% polyunsaturated. Milk fat is a *small* but dependable source of the *essential fatty acids*. These are fatty acids that the body needs for metabolism and which must be derived from the diet since the body is unable to manufacture them. The linoleic acid in milk is in a form which favors the desirable conversion to arachidonic acid.

Milk's emulsified fat is more easily digested than any other food fat except that of eggs. Like other dietary fats, milk fat contributes to the satiety value of a meal and is a concentrated source of energy, providing 50% of whole milk's food energy.

The phospholipids in milk are bound to the surface of the tiny fat globules along with proteins. They are substances containing phophorus, nitrogen and fatty acids.

Cholesterol, the principal sterol in milk fat, makes up about 0.25% of the total fat. Currently there is still much scientific debate about dietary cholesterol, although it is known to be indispensable to the body's normal function. It serves as a precursor for many biologically important steroid sex hormones and much (80%) of the cholesterol metabolized is converted to important bile acids. That's the up-side. On the down-side, cholesterol is a major culprit in the origins of atherosclerosis which leads to heart disease and stroke – the number one cause of death in North America.

The physiological impact of dietary fat and cholesterol is still a subject of heated controversy among scientists and also relates to the desirability of dairy consumption which will also be discussed later.

Carbohydrates

Milk is the only food source of the carbohydrate lactose, although it is the only significant carbohydrate in milk. Some traces of others, such as glucose and glucosamines, are also present. Lactose, a sugar, provides half of the total solids in milk and contributes 30% of the food energy in whole milk.

Lactose has many beneficial characteristics. A relatively low solubility makes it less irritating to the stomach and intestinal mucosa than highly soluble sugars. Lactose stimulates the growth of intestinal micro-organisms that synthesize three B vitamins: biotin, riboflavin and folic acid. It produces organic acids which provide a somewhat protective medium by checking the growth of undesirable bacteria in the intestine. In addition, lactose increases the absorption of calcium, phosphorus and magnesium, and favorably affects the intestinal flora. Cheese and yogurt are low in lactose, as the lactose is converted to lactic acid by the bacterial culture necessary to make these products.

Minerals

Milk contains some of all the minerals known to be needed for good nutrition. Analysis of its mineral ash reveals evidence of calcium, phosphorus, magnesium, potassium, sodium, chlorine, sulphur, and others in trace amounts. Calcium and phosphorus merit particular emphasis.

Think calcium, think milk. That is the effectiveness of the marketing and promotion campaign that the dairy industry continues to wage. It is western dogma, probably more universal in its appeal than any other food claim. The distribution of calcium in popular western foods other than milk and dairy products is not very extensive. It is available in tofu, deep sea fish like sardines and salmon, also in spinach, broccoli, almonds and dried figs, for example. But it is obvious that none of these wins a popularity contest in modern society with its addiction to fast, processed, convenience and junk foods. This could be why studies have revealed that calcium, such an essential nutrient, is often lacking in the Western diet. The calcium in milk is readily available for utilization by the body because it is highly dispersed in the ionic form essential for absorption. The lactose present further favors this calcium absorption.

However, there is a real paradox. As we mentioned, calcium is essential for normal bones and teeth; it also functions as a catalyst in several enzymatic reactions and affects nerve and muscle performance. But interestingly enough, the major widespread consequence of calcium deficiency seen later in life (osteoporosis) is *not* more prevalent in areas where milk and dairy products are not abundant in the diet. The issues are therefore much more complex and we will come back to this also, a little later in this chapter.

Milk also contains phosphorus in a readily utilized form and, in the calcium to phosphorus ratio, it is ideal for body use. There is an interdependence of calcium, phosphorus and vitamin D in the body, and all should be available simultaneously for efficient utilization. All three nutrients are involved in, and are essential for, normal bone and tooth formation. Milk fortified with vitamin D is designed to deliver results.

Vitamins

Whole milk also contains some of all the vitamins known to be required by man. These include the fat-soluble vitamins A, E and K which are found in the fat phase of milk. Whole milk contains significant amounts of vitamin A and its fat-soluble precursor, carotene, that imparts its creamy color. When fat is removed (as in 2% or skim milk), the vitamin A content decreases accordingly. The Food and Drug Regulations require the addition of vitamin A to all skim and partly-skimmed milks within the range of 1200 - 2500 IU for each quart (946 ml). Then, as we noted above, vitamin D is needed for the body's utilization of calcium and phosphorus. Most non-dairy foods are also poor sources of vitamin D. Since milk is a common food consumed in North America, it was selected to be fortified. The Food and Drug Regulations require the addition of 300-400 IU of vitamin D per quart of milk. The vitamin D added is usually in the molecular form of cholecalciferol (D3). Finally, both vitamin E, an antioxidant that prevents fat oxidation, and vitamin K, which is involved in blood clotting, are found in very small amounts in whole milk.

Milk in its liquid phase also contains the water-soluble vitamins: ascorbic acid (vitamin C) and the eight essential B-vitamins group. Since they are synthesized by micro-organisms in the rumen of the dairy cow, their concentration in milk remains fairly constant. Milk is an excellent source of *riboflavin*. Little of this valuable nutrient is lost through pasteurization since it is stable to heat. But it can be destroyed by ultraviolet light so these losses are prevented by the use of opaque milk cartons and of course, darkened refrigerators. Although milk appears to provide a low level of *niacin* (nicotinic acid), it is a good source of the amino acid tryptophan, which can be converted to niacin in the body, thereby giving milk a high niacin equivalent. Milk also contains significant amounts of the heat labile B vitamin, *thiamin*. Its losses during pasteurization, drying and condensing can be minimal when modern techniques are used.

Milk provides small amounts of the other B vitamins. *Pyridoxine* (B6) occurs in milk as pyridoxal, a biologically active agent. Essential for amino acid metabolism, it acts as a co-enzyme in transamination and in the conversion of tryptophan to niacin. *Pantothenic acid* (another B-vitamin) is relatively stable in moist heat and little is lost during pasteurization. It is essential for all living organisms and is a constituent of Co-enzyme A. Similarly, *folacin (folic acid)*, necessary for normal blood and fetal neural tube formation, is found in very small amounts in milk. However, milk is one of the best sources of *cyanocobalamin* (B12), a vitamin directly related to the prevention of pernicious anemia; it is found only in foods of animal origin. Milk is considered a good source of *biotin* (even though it has only minute quantities) since only 40mg are needed each day to supplement that synthesized in the intestine. Choline, which is involved in synthesis of a neurotransmitter and in fat transport in the body, and inositol, which may also be involved, are both also found in milk.

However, milk is not a major source of the other critical water-soluble vitamin, C. In order to meet the needs of formula-fed infants who do not receive citrus fruit juice, the Food and Drug Regulations require the addition of vitamin C to evaporated milk.

THE OTHER SIDE OF MILK

Clearly, from the above discussion, milk (and dairy products, in general) does appear to be a very nutritious food, readily available from a *natural* source, and well accepted in Western society. Many people buy cow's milk regularly for their families, based on the popular ideas that this product provides essential nutrients like calcium and protein, that it helps to build healthy bodies, and that indeed, the family's precious health would be in jeopardy if they did not drink of nature's wholesome goodness…this nutritious beverage we call milk.

But is that the complete picture?

No, it certainly is not. In more recent time, many students of human nutrition, an increasing number of pediatricians and other doctors who see health consequences associated with regular milk consumption, an increasing number of natural health and wellness advocates, and many consumer advocates, all join in voices of protest against the deleterious effects of cow's milk in the North American diet. They question the advertising claims, they are suspicious of the dairy lobby and its research funding, and they distrust the nutrition establishment.

But this is not a question for activism per se. It is a case for good research and a matter of science. And scientists have responded on both sides of the 'Milk Divide'. The establishment is clearly still on the side of the dairy industry and its protagonists. Conventional dieticians and nutritionists still sing the praises of cow's milk as 'essential, if not ideal food' and an excellent source of good human nutrition. Milk is a common inclusion in school lunches and hospital meals. Advertisers promote its virtue, politicians vote for its financial backing and many doctors recommend its regular use. But, that is the orthodox tradition.

More recently, several reputable physicians and nutritionists have questioned the basic premises regarding cow's milk. They have examined the evidence and come to the somewhat surprising conclusion that the case against the regular consumption of cow's milk across the board is strong and even compelling. Some now caution against the use of cow's milk for specific groups or in specific circumstances; others are equivocal about its net value in the diet in general; and a vocal but disorganized lobby group adamantly opposes its use by humans altogether. They think cow's milk presents a real hazard to health and should be better regarded as a deadly poison.

The dissent is not from some lunatic fringe of the medical or scientific community. For example, more than a decade ago, the Committee on Nutrition of the prestigious American Academy of Pediatrics (the institutional voice of all the practicing American pediatricians) released a comprehensive report (1983) with the provocative title: *"Should Milk Drinking by Children Be Discouraged?"* The academy is still apprehensive (as of now) and gives a qualified 'maybe' as an answer. But the surprise is that this question was even raised in the first place. Especially in that group.

A much stronger position against cow's milk was taken by the eminent Pediatrician, Dr. Frank Oski, one time Director of the Department of Pediatrics at St. John's Hopkins University School of Medicine and Physician-in-Chief of the John Hopkins Children's Center. He is a contributing author or editor to no less than 19 medical textbooks and 290 medical manuscripts. He wrote a little classic entitled *"Don't drink your Milk!"* in which the message is clear. Dr. Oski pointed out that "the drinking of cow's milk has been linked to iron-deficiency anemia in infants and children; it has been named as the cause of cramps and diarrhea in much of the world's population, and the cause of multiple forms of allergy as well; and the possibility has been raised that it may play a central role in the origin of atherosclerosis and heart attacks." That's big league stuff.

Dr. William Ellis, a retired osteopathic physician and surgeon from Texas, researched the health effects of dairy products for more than forty years. This highly regarded osteopath concluded that cow's milk and other dairy products were "simply no good for humans". He became convinced of the "overwhelming evidence that milk and milk products are harmful to many people, both adults and infants. Milk is a contributing factor in constipation, chronic fatigue, arthritis, headaches, muscle cramps, obesity, allergies and heart problems". Even the late Dr. Benjamin Spock, the world-famous pediatrician, advocated in 1992 the avoidance of cow's milk for babies and infants. He was particularly concerned about the incidence of milk-derived allergy and colic in the little ones. Many other voices have been raised in opposition to the most effective dairy industry propaganda and some of the research must out of necessity be included here.

Even a cursory review of the thousands of medical abstracts related to the clinical impact of cow's milk would reveal that it does not get a high evaluation or recommendation at least in the technical literature. It is not seen as a "perfect food". Rather, the main focus of published research seems to be on associated problems like intestinal colic, irritation and bleeding, anemia and allergic reactions in infants and children. In adults, the issues revolve around heart disease, arthritis, and the more serious possibility of affecting leukemia, lymphoma and other cancers. There is an ominous fear of potential viral infection with bovine leukemia virus, if for some reason or fluke, the normally effective pasteurization did not kill it where it does exist. There is discussion regarding contamination with infected cells, and a variety of chemicals, insecticides and other toxins.

Much of this is the exceptional rather than the general observation, often more theoretical than realistic, and based more on principle than in practice. But there are many such undesirable side effects of cow's milk consumption which are by no means infrequent, and there are several real contraindications. This is balanced only by the purported benefit of milk calcium and vitamin D ingestion to protect against osteoporosis, and the contribution to the daily requirements for complete and balanced protein. In more recent time, there have been some research reports that also support a protective influence of milk consumption against colorectal cancers, and against even kidney stones and stroke.

Just the composition of cow's milk relative to human milk should raise some questions. When compared to human mother's milk, cow's milk is about three times richer in protein and five to seven times richer in minerals, while being very deficient in essential fatty acids. The cow's milk is designed for a young calf with its need for massive skeletal growth and huge muscle groups. Hence, it is dense in protein and calories as fat. In contrast, humans are distinguished by marked specialization. Human infants take about six months to double their relatively small birth weight and so human milk is low in protein. Calves, on the other hand, require only a month and a half to double their birth weight, so cow's milk is richer in protein. Plus, the nature of the protein is quite different. Cow's milk has twenty times as much casein as human milk, making it less digestible for humans. Therefore, a tendency to poorly digested protein could cause problems in the gut. It may be associated with fairly widespread milk protein allergy and it could have possible impact on the immune system.

Earlier in this chapter, we made the case briefly for the nutritious value of milk, and throughout the lifecycle. There is clearly some value there. Let's now take a second look at the main nutritional ingredients of milk: calcium, protein, fats and sugar. What follows is the down-side.

Calcium. Most mothers insist that their kids drink their milk because they need its calcium to build those growing bones, healthy and strong. They are convinced that the young people will need calcium to protect against osteoporosis in later life. That's true. The dairy industry is always quick to affirm the copious and convenient supply of calcium in milk and the apparent scarcity of useable calcium elsewhere in the diets of most people in Western countries.

But not so fast. Cow's milk is rich in calcium, yes, but is it a good source for humans?

Dairy protagonists emphasize that the presence of calcium in milk as salts (calcium caseinate and calcium phosphate) makes the highly dispersed ionic form convenient for absorption. They further point out the synergy with the intrinsic lactose and the vitamin D participation. Those facts score points for milk.

But opponents insist that the calcium in milk is not easily absorbed, for two reasons, first, calcium is partly bound to protein which inhibits absorption. Secondly, the high protein concentration in milk makes it quite acidic so the blood has to be therefore neutralized by absorbing alkaline minerals including calcium from the bone. This is regulated by the hormone thyrocalcitonin and which in turn, further inhibits absorption.

A number of studies have found that vegetarians have much stronger bones than high-protein meat eaters. By age 65, meat eaters have five to six times as much measurable bone loss as vegetarians. A study in the U.S. actually showed a worsening in calcium balance in post-menopausal women given three 8-ounce glasses of cows' milk per day. The critically important effects (other than calcium) are related to hormones (estrogen), gender, weight bearing on axial bones and in particular, protein intake. To further demonstrate that the cow's milk is not the important source of dietary calcium, there are no recorded dietary deficiencies of calcium among people living on a natural diet without milk. Eskimos for example, have an exceptionally high intake of protein (estimated at 25 percent of total calories) and of calcium (2,500mg/day). Yet their osteoporosis is among the worst in the world. In contrast, the Bantus of South Africa have only a 12 percent protein diet, mainly from plants, and a mere 200-300mg/day of calcium, about half to one third that of North Americans. Yet their women have virtually no osteoporosis despite bearing several children and nursing them extensively. The *piece de resistance* is that when these African women migrate to the U.S., they do develop osteoporosis, though not quite as much as Caucasian or Asian women. All this suggests a role for both genetics and diet, and possibly other factors too.

So where else could one obtain calcium? Just think of it. Where do cows get calcium? From eating the green plants that extract it from the soil; there's another big plus for green, leafy vegetables. That's how the other half of the world lives – no cow's milk, but just lots of greens! That's how animals in the wild build their strong bones. As Robert M. Kradjan M.D., observed in an open letter to his patients, "only humans living an affluent lifestyle have rampant osteoporosis."

There is a better way, but that must await a new development discussed in Chapter Ten.

Protein.   It was perhaps only until a generation ago that nutritionists and dietitians were emphasizing the need for adequate, complete and balanced protein. The more we learned of molecular biology, DNA and protein synthesis, the more important proteins appeared. So the corollary was to get that protein in. Supply nature with the amino acid building blocks and genetics would do the rest. That made sense.

It made sense until we began to realize that there were implications. Excess nitrogen was a burden on the kidneys. Protein was usually not alone but often accompanied in the diet by the new culprits: cholesterol and fat. So the Recommended Dietary Allowances (RDA's in the U.S.) and Recommended Daily Nutrient Intake (RDNI's in Canada) were steadily revised downward. The current recommendation is as low as 0.75gm/kilo/day for adults 19 through 51 years. So the typical 70kg male (who's that, disregarding our obese culture?) would require a mere 50-55 grams of protein each day. And that's generous. The World Health Organization has estimated the real need to be only 0.6gm/kilo/day. That means 40-45 grams of protein for the stereotype adult.

One ounce and a half, that's all! Most adults drinking milk as a staple beverage are living with a protein overload. A single cup (240ml) of whole milk contains 8.5 grams of protein and 26 percent of the Daily Value for saturated fat. One could consider milk a kind of "liquid meat" as far as protein intake goes.

Vegetable proteins, particularly soya beans and its derivatives, are excellent sources of protein and with good variety, there is little justifiable concern about imbalance or amino acid deficiency. There is no intrinsic need for protein derived uniquely from meat or dairy. On the contrary, one has to be vigilant regarding excess intake and with the associated high fat, high cholesterol accompaniment. These dangers are well known in our media culture where cardiovascular disease is the number one cause of death. The Heart and Stroke Foundation will not allow us to forget. They should not.

Milk Fats (Lipids).   However you put it, the high fat content in whole milk from cows can only be detrimental at a time when cardiovascular disease and cancer are the leading causes of death in society. Add in the cholesterol content and you have a recipe for an unhealthy food beverage.   To dairy detractors, it's as simple as that. Milk is a major contributor of saturated fat in the adult North American diet. Only cheese and beef contribute more. The public knows this now and there is a marked trend toward the consumption of more low fat dairy products. In the past three decades, there has been a 50 percent decline in milk fat consumption from milk itself, but that has been more than offset by a huge increase in consumption of milk fat from cheese. Therefore between 1970 and 1994 the per capita availability of total dietary milk fat actually rose by 4 per cent.

There is now a good consensus among the lipid experts, including both nutritionists and clinicians, that the healthy diet today should contain no more than 30 percent of total calories as fat and 10 percent as saturated fat. Even low fat milk contains as much as 24 to 33% calories as fat. The designation of 2% milk is misleading to the public since it refers to 2% by weight, when milk is 87% water by weight. Remove the water content and the real picture comes to light. Whole milk is even worse. The debate is virtually over with respect to dietary fat and cholesterol. Almost all health professionals today would agree that diets high in fat and cholesterol promote cardiovascular disease and several cancers including possibly ovary, breast and prostate.

Speaking of cancers, just consider the following results from three related studies conducted at the Roswell Park Memorial Institute in Buffalo, New York (1989):

1. The beverage habits of 569 lung cancer patients and an equal number of controls were studied. Persons drinking whole milk 3 or more times daily had a 5-fold increase in lung cancer risk when compared to those never drinking whole milk.
2. The diets of 371 prostate cancer patients and comparable control subjects were examined. Men who reported drinking 3 or more glasses of whole milk daily had a relative risk of 2.49 compared with men who reported never drinking whole milk.
3. Drinking more than one glass of whole milk or equivalent daily, gave a woman a 3.1 times increased risk of ovarian cancer over non-milk users.

These results are typical of the type of epidemiological data found for the relative risk of both cancer and cardiovascular disease with respect to high fat diets in general, and whole milk consumption in particular. Whatever the true disease association, prudence would suggest an increased shift on the part of wise consumers away from whole milk, just from a consideration of reducing dietary fat.

Lactose (Milk Sugar). The principal carbohydrate in milk you recall, is a dissacharide sugar called lactose. This molecule is too large for absorption in the intestine, it is first broken down by the action of enzymes, including the major one lactase, into galactose and glucose which are then absorbed. Lactase is generally present in the gut in early childhood and then declines with age. By age 4 or 5, most of the world population is no longer equipped to handle **lactose** in the diet. This is a normal, natural process of maturation and development. Could nature be saying something? When the enzyme is not effective, lactose remains in the gut to be broken down by bacterial fermentation, producing acids, carbon dioxide and hydrogen gas. These lead to the common symptoms associated with lactose intolerance, namely diarrhea, gas and abdominal cramps.

There is a clear genetic predisposition to this lactose intolerance: blacks have up to 90%, Caucasians about 20-40%, and Orientals somewhere in the middle. There is now a commercial source of the lactase enzyme (Lactaid™ tablets or drops). Lactese™ is a special milk made available with low lactose content for those who wish to drink milk despite their lactose intolerance. Of course, lactose-free soy milk is a simple, natural alternative in this regard.

NATURE CALLS FOR SCIENCE

So what's the jury's verdict? Is milk a panacea for human nutrition with all its rich ingredients? Or does milk pose a threat to human health? Should it be universally promoted to people of all ages for their health and benefit, or should it carry warning labels?

This jury declares a mis-trial. All the evidence has not been discovered. Cow's milk is ubiquitous in the Western world, the product of a vast dairy industry and a staple food for many years. Clearly, it has much to offer as part of an adequate, balanced diet to satisfy real human nutrient requirements. But at the same tine, milk is a package with ingredients that prove undesirable and sometimes unhealthy. This risk to benefit analysis calls for more empirical science to discriminate. Unless we subject every ingredient to analysis and the complete dairy products to epidemiology and clinical assessment, it is impossible to draw any valid conclusions for universal application.

The dairy establishment has led the public at large to rush to judgement but it is time for second opinion, a re-assessment based on further scientific inquiry. Like Sherlock Holmes, we have to pursue the facts, just the plain facts. These facts are ascertained by empirical analysis where objective minds make careful observations and rational deductions.

Milk is a natural product. All natural products deserve the scrutiny of science. **Only such a union of the best of nature and the best of science can give birth to the best of human health**. In the next chapter we will explore this emerging relationship. Later we will discover buried in this goldmine, far more than we plan for.

Chapter Three

NATURE & SCIENCE
Making The Connection

I choose to begin this chapter with a personal anecdote that illustrates why it is so important to be wise, responsible and diligent in the pursuit of health and wellness, even when one pursues the *natural route* alternative.

My family's roots can be traced back for two hundred years in the tiny islands of the Caribbean. A European landowner way back there fathered a child with a black slave woman and three generations later, my mother was born. With her stronger African genes, she was predisposed to hypertension and showed symptoms of this disease at an early age. I was born when mother was only thirty two and I only knew her with elevated blood pressures. As a primary school teacher, and a mother of six, she was a very active, hardworking woman. Her blood pressure would go up and down and so would her capacity to function. When it was really up, and it seemed to be like that so often, she would be confined to home with massive headaches and fatigue. Our brilliant family doctors made house calls over the years and took great care of her with their limited pharmacotherapy. We watched her endure this malignant form of the terrible hypertensive disease and despite her courage, her faith and her determination, this loving saint we called 'mother' succumbed to her condition and had a fatal cerebral hemorrhage at the young and tender age of forty nine.

But why this personal anecdote?

The fact is that in the islands, a tradition had developed sur-rounding a common *natural* plant called *periwinkle*. It is sometimes called wintergreen or myrtle but it belongs to the *Apocynaceae* family and has the scientific name, *Vinca minor*. In any case, it was popularly believed in the islands, that this plant was 'good for high blood pres-sure' and so, just as you would imagine, it was common to pick the leaves and stems to boil in water to make this therapeutic tea.

I recall many a day, and a late night too, that we would anx-iously collect our 'special periwinkle select' and prepare a heart-warm-ing brew for mother. The more sick she was, the more she would need of this so-called 'lifesaver.' And so the more eagerly and lovingly, we would serve her this natural *remedy for her ills.*

But that periwinkle tea was a toxic portion in disguise. Natu-ral-products chemists have had a curiosity about this periwinkle plant since it has been used traditionally for more than hypertension. In the absence of science, nature can run wild and she often does. Trial and error leads to mis-association and often false claims. There are no reli-able criteria.

In the world of 'natural remedies', periwinkle is used for "brain health" which translates to increasing cerebral circulation, supporting brain metabolism, increasing mental productivity, preventing memory and concentration impairment and feebleness, improving memory and thinking capacity, preventing premature aging of brain cells and geriat-ric support. It is also used for mucous membrane inflammation, diar-rhea, vaginal discharge, "blood purification", throat ailments, tonsilli-tis, angina, sore throat, intestinal inflammation, toothache, edema, pro-moting wound healing, improving immune function, and as a diuretic, sedative, hemostatic remedy, and a bitter.

Clearly, like most well-established natural products, a lot of *folklore* had evolved around the supposed benefits of this common plant. The range of ailments for which it was reputed to have some therapeutic value was so diverse, that to hazard a guess at any common mechanism of action would have been difficult. Grandparents and their grandpar-ents have testified to periwinkle's efficacy. That's the traditional value of this *natural* alternative. No wonder the analytical chemists pursued the facts.

What did they find?

The same periwinkle plant is now known to contain pharmacologically active, toxic alkaloids that can cause nerve, liver and kidney damage. These include, for example, *vincristine* which has definite cytotoxic and neurological actions and is used in anti-cancer drug cocktails. One constituent, *vincamine*, does have hypotensive activity. But that is only a small part of the total package. It may even have been an effective and in some circumstances, an attractive part of the complete picture. But in animals, periwinkle causes leukocytopenia, lymphocytopenia, and lowers alpha-1, alpha-2, and gamma-globulin levels, presumably due to immune suppression.

The periwinkle tea that we served mother was indeed, probably unsafe at best and only the love with which it was served could compensate for the possible toxic consequences.

And what's the bottom line? Periwinkle has since been declared **unsafe for human consumption** by the U.S. FDA due to the known constituent alkaloids and should now be avoided.

The fact is that because something is *natural* does not necessarily imply that it is either good for your health or that it is primarily safe. There are poisons in nature. Some have immediate effects – they cause acute illness or even death – and the word soon spreads that those are to be avoided. Others may be more slow in their devastation, but the cumulative effects eventually take hold. The subtlety of the damage and therefore the health risk, may remain obscure for centuries until more careful observation and analysis bring the disappointing truth to light.

But tradition has a life of its own.

Anecdotes are not enough

With the rise in popularity of alternative medicine, a vast array of *natural* products and therapeutic procedures have come to market. Some of these were reviewed in Chapter One. But that's only the tip of the iceberg that we looked at. It seems as though every few weeks or months, there is some media report or advertising blitz promoting the virtue of some new panacea. There are claims and counter-claims. And in the age of the effective sound-bite, there is nothing like a credible and convincing testimonial. Infomercials on daily television make a collage of such first-hand experiences of presumably real-people, in homely settings, that are supposed to authenticate the product or procedure being essentially advertised. It's direct and 'in-your-face.' The message is, 'it did it for me, it will do the same for you.'

There is no way to distinguish by mere listening, who's real or who's just acting a part; who's telling the truth or simply making it up. But the advertisers know that the masses are gullible. Say it on television or radio, write it up in the newspapers or magazines, or just put out a flyer, especially with pictures of real people – and some people will inevitably believe. After all, the public now wants to believe. We want simple, *natural* solutions.

And so the stories are told. No questions asked. The cancer patient had tried everything and in desperation turned to some special remedy and *voilà*, the cancer is gone ... The spouse could never avoid snoring, so the partner had moved to another bedroom – then they came across the solution – it worked! And then they're sleeping together again ... The weight-loss industry keeps rolling along with the latest fad diet and real-life *before and after* pictures to demonstrate what you could potentially look like ... and the beat goes on. One anecdote after another, as if health and vitality were obtained just like cleaning one's laundry.

But it does not come that way.

Just think of it. Even if you allow that individual health testimonials are truly honest and complete, how would that justify making generalizations for society at large. After all, we are a collection of all unique individuals. No two of us are identical - not even identical twins who have different life experiences and exposures after birth. The rest of us have different genes, different environments, different lifestyles, different experiences, different medical histories, different idiosyncrasies, and so on, and so on. It is foolhardy to presume in the area of health and wellness that if any one person, or even any random group of people, have a specific experience or result with the use of any given product or procedure, that the same is to be expected for any other person or group. There are just too many variables! Individual experiences and anecdotes are not enough. 'One man's meat is another man's poison.' Yes, even as *natural* a thing as meat.

Yet so much of the alternative natural foods and natural therapies continue to be promoted in this anecdotal way. We see it everywhere, in all forms of advertising. And as in all advertising, there is the latent power of association. So the anecdotes assume new authority and persuasion if they are related to us by some media celebrity. Promoters have even been known to *buy* the endorsement of professionals who add their credentials to the quoted anecdotes for some given natural alternative. But that does not change the facts. The more one can hype the story, dramatize the result, exaggerate the claim and promise relief and benefit, the more the market responds. It is the alternative way. By its very methodology, it goes against the establishment with its orthodoxy. It opens new frontiers and possibilities. Best of all, it offers hope. Hopefully, not something else in disguise.

In one sense, this experience-based health and wellness dogma has been a secret to the success of the entire alternative, self-help, natural products movement. It has become its *modus operandi*. It gets the message out quickly and effectively, and at little cost. The same story lights a spark and when it is repeated often, sometimes it spreads like a prairie fire on a windy day. And that metaphor is appropriate for in some cases, it can do harm and cause devastation in its course. It has at times, hurt its own cause. What disservice has been done because so many have been gullible to anecdotal reports and put themselves at risk. What consequences have followed the inappropriate use of the unproven *natural* therapies and panaceas that could not deliver what they promised.

But some of the *natural* purists would argue that time is the ultimate test of efficacy, safety and value. They contend that if a natural product has been used for centuries (sometimes millenia), and still finds a place in common remedies with associated claims, then the ultimate proof of real worth is its longevity. It sounds almost like a true *natural selection* process. Food, for example, has been around from the dawn of civilization but nutrition is still in its infancy. The safety and benefit of different plants, fish and lower animals have been derived from the results of experience, not from nutritionists and scientists in laboratories. Some things were edible and some were not. The test of each was in the eating. Our early ancestors were so-called guinea pigs (to mix a metaphor technically) and unfortunately some did not live long enough even to tell the tale. But their neighbors and friends learnt from their experiments each time and so learnt what to eat and what not to eat. Similarly, the use of traditional herbs for therapeutic value and the practice of traditional healing arts have withstood the test of time and therefore, it is argued, they remain invincible. In the absence of anything more or any better alternative, that argument would suffice. But there is a better way. It's called *science*!

Before we pursue this interesting relationship between nature and science, let's just consider a more sophisticated and reliable form of this traditional anecdotal experience. Today, it's called a Case Report.

Case Reports

The medical and scientific literature is filled with published Case Reports. Many journals have reserved pages for reporting of unusual or remarkable individual observations that warrant dissemination to the professional community. There are even publications devoted almost exclusively to Case Reports. Sometimes, to expedite reporting, the author(s) may write a letter to the journal editors for fast communication.

But a published Case Report is much more than just anther anecdote. At least in three ways. First, Case Reports are based on careful, thorough observations by a third party. It is not a subjective recollection of some effect or experience that is so vague or general that it poses more questions than it answers. The author is usually a professional with credentials that attest to some reliable powers of observation in a clinical or somewhat controlled setting. The observation might be random or unprovoked but the circumstances are carefully documented and wherever possible, the results are quantitative or at least well-characterised.

Secondly, a Case Report is usually made within defined parameters. Care is taken to identify all influential factors, to avoid confounding variables which would make conclusions meaningless, and where possible, to negate the obvious placebo effect or null solution. A good Case Report is always a detailed report not simply a conclusion that is desirable. Generally, the subject in question is not manipulated by controlled variables, as in the laboratory or even in a designed experimental study in the field. But the observations are made nevertheless in confined circumstances. The case is not general, it is particular. The details are unique to this set of circumstances, but they provoke further questions and point in new directions of understanding.

That brings us to the third and perhaps most important difference between a simple anecdotal experience that promoters of *natural alternatives* so commonly use, and the more formal published Case Report. It has to do with the intent and application of the reported result. Case Reports are usually the product of an experience by default rather than by design. There is no presumed agenda, no attempt to build a case or prove a point. It simply reports an interesting or unusual observation. There's almost an element of surprise. Such genuine Case Reports are never recorded as general prescriptions for widespread or universal application. They are not intended to make an argument for any particular course of action. Unlike so many testimonials, they are the beginning of inquiry and not the end. They initiate more research rather than avoid or preclude it. Clearly, the value of Case Reports is that they encourage questions, they stimulate hypotheses, they generate new experiments – in a word, they advance the cause of good science.

Which leads us to that all important relationship between nature and science.

Nature and Science

Primitive man (read generically, male and female) was a curious man. Intrigued by the world around him and by his own nature, he set about to learn by trial and error. It may have taken a long time, but despite the odds, primitive tools were discovered, and so were fire combustion and the wheel, etc. But these were incidental findings with unsophisticated deductive reasoning. Later, the Ancient Greeks and Romans as well as the early Egyptians showed genuine curiosity about the world around them and cultivated their minds with fundamentals of mathematics, philosophy and the like. However, when Constantinople entrenched Christianity in the known world, the anti-intellectuals took over. They burned the libraries of their time and plunged the human civilization into the Dark Ages. Some historians believe that it was the rise of Islam with a strong emphasis on individual enlightenment and a prescribed social order, that caused the beginning of a return to inquiry and scholarship leading to the Age of Enlightenment. Yet nature remained so much of an enigma with unanswered philosophical questions while research, for what it was, stumbled along. Then elitism and tradition imposed a sterile inertia of thought and reason in the orthodox Roman church and therefore much of the known world. There was nothing apparent to research but esoteric theology, and there was no one equipped to even begin the process of research but the clerical mystics trapped in their self-spun transcendental contemplations. The manipulation of ordinary laity and attendant corruption took over. Dogma replaced discussion.

But nature continued to pose a challenge and a threat to sterile orthodoxy. Changes in nature ... from the daily rising and setting of the sun, the night sky, or the simple evaporation and condensation of water ... cried out for further investigation. However, darkness covered the minds of humanity while superstition and corrupt theology strangled any initiative to free inquiry. Thus it remained for hundreds of years.

Then came the awakening of a young German monk called Martin Luther, who penetrated the darkness of the sixteenth century. A new revelation captured his mind and spirit which soon spread to John Calvin, John Knox and a line of Protestant Reformers who shook the establishment with bold new affirmations of a free and renewed theology. They gained a liberating understanding of the Divine essence, His nature and will. They came to affirm His creative presence in His creation and most of all His initiative in *revelation*. Suddenly these reformers could discern the handiwork of a consistent First Cause and the direct and permissive will of the Unmoved Mover. He was not capricious; He was faithful in all his works from the beginning. These same works could be "sought out by all those who took pleasure therein." Yes, any individual who was willing to pursue truth, could find it. It could be personal, but not particular to that individual. Something real and objective was there for all to know, by empirical means.

With this new theology, modern science was born. Then came a line of true researchers, in pursuit of universal laws which were directed and controlled by the Law Maker and the Law Giver. He was willing and even anxious to reveal Himself in creation, *in nature*, in history just as much as in the Holy Scriptures or the Church.

Suddenly there was no longer mutual exclusivity between faith and reason; no easy capitulation to fatalism and chance. Now it was clear that there was no inherent contradiction between the Creator and His creation; no need for blind obedience to imposed dogma. Nature stood apart from the mind but was subject to the reasoning of the mind. **There was an objective reality that was worth investigating. It was reproducible and predictable. Experimental inquiry could be the route to natural revelation.**

So modern science took root and began to grow.

At the heart of this new pursuit was the *a priori* conviction of the universality of natural causes. There was a consistency of cause and effect. The immutability of the Uncaused Cause made every other cause to lead necessarily to a definite and specific effect. Therefore, experimental results were predictable. All observed phenomena, whether natural or controlled, even in different hands, at different times and places, with different sample materials, would all yield the same, consistent results. Phenomena could be understood and once the underlying *laws* or *principles* were discovered, new phenomena could be predicted. Yes, nature could be explained by this new science and moreover, it could be changed. For the better or for the worse becomes a moral and ethical question, but nature could now be exploited one way or the other. In the past three hundred years, science and technology have since been used to change the world beyond recognition. That has been sometimes for the better, but sadly, sometimes for the worse too.

Yet we must remember that despite all the technological achievements, we don't know how to make a single blade of grass. One wiser than Solomon himself pointed out that "even Solomon, in all his glory, was not arrayed like one of these (lilies of the field)." As Prince Charles wisely remarked in his Millenium Reith lecture recently:

"Faced with such unknowns, it is hard not to feel a sense of humility, wonder and awe about our place in the natural order."

He further admonished us to *"show greater respect for the genius of nature's designs, rigorously tested and refined over millions of years. This means being careful to use science to understand how nature works, not to change essentially what nature is, as we do when genetic manipulation seeks to transform a process of biological evolution into something altogether different. The idea that the different parts of the natural world are connected through an intricate system of checks and balances, which we disturb at our peril, is all too easily dismissed as no longer relevant."*

And so the question is never to be one of contradistinction, that is between science *or* nature. It must be an appropriate combination of science *and* nature. In our contemporary world, the best of nature must unite with the best of science to harvest and harness all that is available from the world of nature, all for the benefit of mankind. To quote Prince Charles again:

"I believe that we need to restore the balance between the heartfelt reason of instinctive wisdom and the rational insights of scientific analysis. Neither, I believe, is much use on its own."

I agree. **The movement to rediscover the traditional value in ancient herbs, natural foods and alternative therapies cannot sacrifice the scrutiny of scientific analysis in the name of Nature.** No one can presume the right to proselytize or prescribe to vulnerable or suffering human beings, in search of better health, even the most natural solution, without some fundamental scientific credibility. That would be unwarranted, irresponsible and downright dangerous.

The call then, is for the scientific method.

The Scientific Method

The basic principles of the scientific method have now become standard in almost every field of human inquiry. Science itself is objective study of natural phenomena. But in the modern world, science has earned the ultimate authoritative role by virtue of the outstanding human achievement it has made possible. The rigorous approach is now considered the *open* door to reality. (Some mistakenly think it is the *only* door, but we will address that later.)

The scientific method is the process of objectively analyzing phenomena and drawing logical conclusions. It is a structured procedure that scientists use to develop theories and laws about the universe. It is all based on observation. Science cannot truly deal with anything that cannot be observed. But that itself poses the inherent problem –

namely, there is a limit and imperfection to the sensory perceptions of the observer. Thus, although the scientific method and the tools of science are powerful tools of knowledge, there are limits to its applicability and certainty.

The procedure or process that is generally called the scientific method may be illustrated as in Fig. 1. In a classical case, something prompts a question to the inquiring mind. It may be an initial observation of an event, or a set of given data, or a mathematical construct or simply an imaginative idea. In any case, a question is asked which prompts an initial reasonable hypothesis. This hypothesis becomes a starting point which allows the design of an experiment.

Figure 1. The Scientific Method

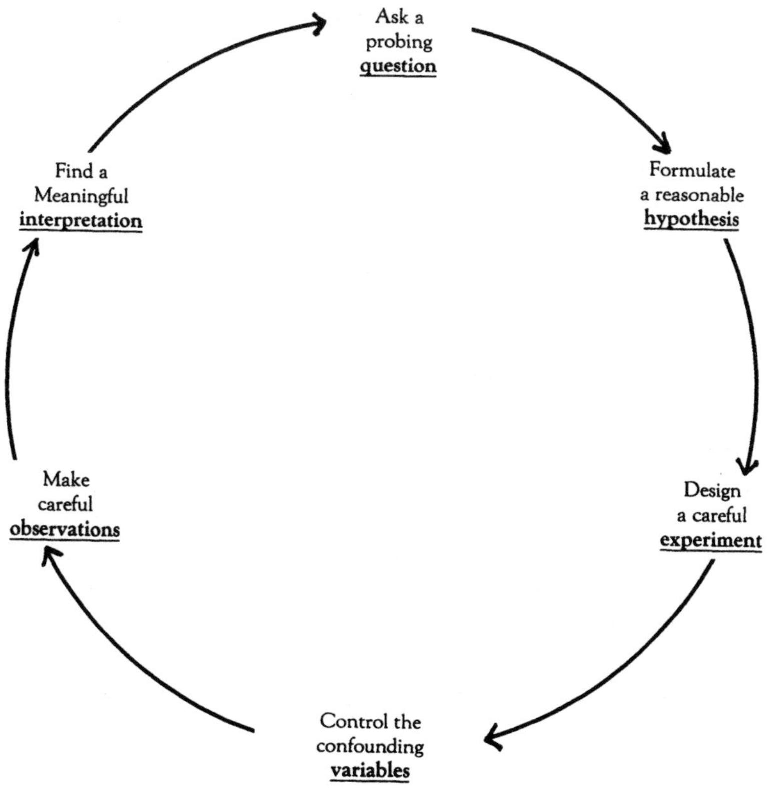

Ask a probing **question**

Formulate a reasonable **hypothesis**

Design a careful **experiment**

Control the confounding **variables**

Make careful **observations**

Find a Meaningful **interpretation**

On the basis of this initial hypothesis, an experiment is logically deduced that will predictably result in a set of particular observations that should occur, under particular conditions, if the hypothesis is true. The experiment is conducted with care to control as many variables as possible in order to define probable cause and effect relationships. The more responsible and consistent the observations, the more positive predictive value of the hypothesis, the stronger the hypothesis will be. All the observations must find meaningful interpretation. If all the particular observations of the designed experiment concur with those predicted by the hypothesis, then the hypothesis is accepted as true. When the hypothesis is substantiated through repeated extensive testing, it becomes an accepted theory or law in the scientific community and is treated as fact. If the observations from experiment do not agree with the hypothesis, then the hypothesis must be revised, the experiment re-examined for uncontrolled variables or the analysis of the results revamped. The new, revised hypothesis then starts the cycle all over again.

But there are many pitfalls, especially in interpretation of experimental data. A correlation between two things does not prove that one thing causes the other. After all, the second thing could even cause the first or some other underlying factor or influence could cause the correlation. Therefore, it is always important to rule out all other possible underlying factors before coming to conclusions of cause and effect. Although scientific proofs cannot be known with absolute certainty, enough evidence can, in principle, be accumulated to be reasonably certain. At least, within defined limits. As the boundaries change, theories can be, and often are, revised.

Scientism

But is that all there is? You may ask that question. Is there nothing more than cold, rational thought and empirical observation. Even if that answered all the *how* questions, what about the *why*? Scientists in the philosophical tradition of positivism would respond that the *why* questions are for the theologians and philosophers, not the scientists. So many of them are materialists who would only acknowledge the existence of concrete material things, forces and empty space. But the best of modern physics brings all that into serious question and ambiguity. And then there are the idealists who believe that the universe can be best understood by assuming that thought or consciousness is the most fundamental reality. For them, certain mathematical concepts are ideas in the Divine mind, such that any physical reality must conform to these ideas.

Unlike the use of the scientific method as only one mode of reaching a knowledge of truth, scientism claims that science alone can render truth about the real world. Its single-minded adherence to only the empirical, or testable, makes it a strictly scientific worldview, in much the same way that an extreme fundamentalism which rejects science can be seen as a strictly religious worldview. Scientism chooses to do away with all metaphysical, philosophical and religious claims, as the truths they would affirm cannot be apprehended or confirmed by the scientific method. In essence, scientism regards science as the only absolute and justifiable access to the truth.

But it is misguided.

Science, after all, is a human endeavor. It is performed by real human beings and there are many aspects of our humanity that cannot be avoided even in scientific research. (Needless to say, the scientific method would be useless in the arts where the abstractions like music, love, beauty, courage, faith etc are paramount). Some left brain activity can and does even enhance the research process. Any good scientist would confess that he or she witnesses almost daily the role in science of artistic creation and imagination, political manipulation and personal exploitation, wishful thinking, bias, egotism, academic incest, critical review as well as unwarranted criticism, and premature skeptical rejection. The cause of science is still subject to the forces of human nature and culture. Scientists are as trapped by their own intrinsic assumptions and values as anyone else. For the purist, one further comment is warranted here. It is the principle of uncertainty attributed to Heisenberg. He framed it in mathematical terms but it has a simple application. The act of observation requires an impact on nature which changes the aspect of nature observed. So we could never be absolutely sure that what we see is exactly what we think we see, or even that it is present where we thought we saw it. This irreducible uncertainty ultimately keeps us humble in the face of whatever observations we make and whatever conclusions we desire. The more we know, the less certain we become of what we do know.

But the scientific method itself must remain the method of choice in the natural world. It is the only adequate basis for universal prescription in the field of health and wellness.

So, what are the implications?

Clinical Trials

The hallmark of the scientific method applied to medicine and health is the now classical randomized, double-blind clinical trial (RCT). For more than fifty yaers now, clinicians, epidemiologists and statisticians have pooled their expertise to refine this methodology and to demonstrate its validity. The RCT is the best empirical means by which we can establish cause and effect relationships between interventions such as drug therapies or surgical procedures (cause) and variations in symptoms or clinical outcomes (effect).

This is an important principle for it can have major impact on the quality of human life, even in large numbers. It is the rational basis for good decision making and needless to say, there are many unfortunate misadventures of cause and effect that have only lead to morbidity and even death.

To illustrate this, imagine that some new form of sex education is introduced in the high schools of a given community. In the next couple years, there is a dramatic rise observed in venereal disease and teenage pregnancy. One could conclude that sex education caused a rise in both VD and teen pregnancy. But not so fast. These are multifactoral problems. School enrolment could have changed, or the types and lifestyles of the coeds, or the popularity of new influential role models in the media, major change in school policies regarding social influences, and so on. There are certainly many possible variables to produce the observed changes and so correlation does not prove causation. Scientists have to be very careful to rule out all other possible underlying factors before concluding that any one thing *causes* another.

The principle of the RCT is to first establish a group for experimental design. This group will have both inclusive and exclusive criteria so that a number of confounding variables are fixed or eliminated before the trial even begins. The numbers required for a trial can vary but there are statistical methods to determine the significance of any conclusion derived with quantitative levels of confidence. Once the group has been identified, the participants are *randomly* divided into two equivalent subgroups. The intervention to be studied is applied in a different form for each subgroup. One group (the test group) gets the supposedly active form of intervention, whereas the other (so-called *control* group) gets an equivalent and indistinguishable *placebo*. There is no apparent way for the individual participant to know which form of intervention they receive. They are *blind* to the difference. Subsequent observations are made of whatever relevant consequences or outcomes are in question and the data is accumulated. The results are interpreted usually by a third party who also does not know to which subgroup any participant is assigned. They too are *blind* to any differences of intervention. The results are tabulated and finally, the code is broken to see how both subgroups responded by comparison to each other. An important condition is that all members of the initial group in the trial must be accounted for in the subsequent report or publication. It is then eminently reasonable to conclude that the presence of the control group negated other confounding variables, and the difference in outcome was caused by the intervention.

But this double-blind study is too demanding for many *alternative therapy* practitioners. They try to avoid or evade this requirement whenever confronted by other scientists and they offer attempts at rationalization which often constitute mere excuses. They point out that no one will pay for a costly study using low cost natural remedies that cannot be patented or otherwise controlled. That's a fair observation and it does often prove very difficult to initiate this kind of RCT with natural therapies. (With mounting public pressure, governments are now beginning to loosen the purse strings, even if only in a small way, to finance research on the benefits of several *natural* and *alternative* interventions in the health care field. This is certainly as it should be.) Many *alternative* advocates also pretend that people who believe in natural health remedies do not wish to deprive half of any test population (the control group) of assumed health benefits, in order to prove the veracity of what they regard as 'obvious'. That is a weak contention since many more serious RCT's are interrupted when the actual net benefit is proven to be obvious and dramatic. They may even argue that *blind* tests are not possible because of the nature of the intervention. With drugs, a simple pill for example can be readily imitated with a placebo and crossover studies are relatively easy to implement. Natural foods, on the other hand, allow distinction from placebo by sensual taste and smell. True, but this cannot be an insurmountable problem. Many natural products can be appropriately packaged and imitated by placebo.

Promoters of *natural* therapeutic alternatives are also quick to emphasize that most of the early prescription drugs and surgical procedures were introduced without the rigor of RCT screening. Some estimate as much as 80% of common contemporary therapeutics have never been subject to an RCT. It is doubtful that the public would have common access today to the likes of the phenomenal drug Aspirin™, if RCT's were mandatory in the early twentieth century. But that does not negate the necessity today for proper screening for both safety and efficacy of any new proposed therapy. Nature is good, but nature is not all good. **A natural solution is desirable where possible, but it must be demonstrably safe and effective, subject to the same scientific analysis and scrutiny.**

And then there is the question of economics. Indeed, RCT's are expensive, very expensive. Drug companies have a vested interest and the financial muscle to allow them the high cost of R & D, knowing that the high price of prescription drugs will more than compensate. Natural alternatives do not share the same luxury. The mystique or mystery that clouds the nature and origin of a new drug, leaves the consumer in the dark and constrains him/her to pay in ignorance for what he must simply accept without knowledge or understanding. *Natural* products on the other hand, are very ordinary and commonplace, not shrouded in esoterica and the consumer's familiarity precludes any attempts at extortion. So high R & D costs in this case cannot be justified or recovered. Somebody else would have to pay. Yet science must be used to determine what works and what does not, what's worth the expense and risk and what is not. That is the responsible thing to do, sooner or later.

Clinical Trials have become very important in the medical and scientific community. There is now a highly regarded International Society of Clinical Trials which draws together specialists from several disciplines. They have annual meetings and publish their own professional Journal and Newsletter. They elicit papers which discuss RCT design issues, problems arising in the execution of RCT's and many monitoring and data analysis issues. Articles for publication go through the standard peer review process.

Peer Review

Established academic journals are not like the popular press. Articles should appear only after a standard rigorous protocol. There are now thousands of journals published around the world each year and their credibility varies almost like night and day. The most reputable however, are not necessarily the most accurate in terms of reporting the best of scientific research.

The standard procedure is for authors to do their research and submit their draft paper to the journal editor who has a committee that essentially identifies a small group of recognized experts in that particular field. The anonymous draft paper is sent to those experts (referees) for their anonymous rigorous criticism and any positive suggestions for correction, improvement or addition. Their comments go back directly to the editor who in turn, sends them back verbatim to the respective author(s). The author(s) does a point-by-point revision and rebuttal and resubmits to the editor the revised draft which is again sent to the original referees. They again critique the changes, revise their comments and report back anonymously to the editor. This back and forth 'critique and revision' process can continue for months as the authors overcome whatever objections or concerns are raised by the referees. When the editor, supported by an editorial board when necessary, is satisfied that the referees have done their work and the author(s) have met their obligations, a paper is finally accepted for publication.

This entire process from submission of a draft paper, to acceptance, to final publication, can take typically six months to a year or more. That is really the normal process but it is the slow track for scientific communication. Journals often include letters to the editor, printed notes, current communications and so on, where shorter and more urgent results can appear in print, often without peer review. Within any given field however, the specialists usually communicate most rapidly amongst themselves, through frequent academic conferences, publication of abstracts and proceedings, direct dialogue and mail, and most recently, via the Internet.

The Peer Review process is designed to maintain a standard of scientific integrity and to foster true excellence in research. However, it is far from perfect. The reality is, that there are many incestuous relationships among professionals so that behind the scenes, there are breaches of trust and confidentiality and the system is not blind and therefore, not neutral. Egos get in the way. Editorial boards which should maintain the objective standards are often like clubs of indulgent colleagues where pride, position, competition, reputation and even money, do affect many a judgement and decision. Then there is the question of research funding and advertising dollars. Sometimes the referees are obstructionist, lazy, inefficient or careless. Sometimes they pass-on their responsibility for review to other colleagues (of lesser stature) and particularly to their graduate students. Sometimes they turn a deliberate 'blind eye' for obscure reasons. These are just some of the problems that do impact the final outcome. The system is not perfect, it is flawed by human nature, but just like political democracy, it is the best available.

Needless to say, too many erroneous research reports get published even in peer-reviewed journals. But what is more disheartening is that the important scientific information usually reaches the public only when unskilled media personnel pickup some provocative or sensational research summary on the wire services and translates it into a News item in the media. Sometimes, the misinformation can get a life of its own and is instantaneously broadcast around the world before professional comments, sober reflection and any necessary qualifications can be attached to at least provide some balance. Some reports are premature, some are misquoted, some are taken completely out of context, some are actually wrong ... but the media gets its advantage nevertheless and the chips are left to fall where they may. No wonder the thinking public is so skeptical of 'science and medicine in the news.'

Unfortunately, many practitioners who work with the *alternative* and *natural* therapies avoid this Peer Review process altogether. Now specialized journals, newsletters, magazines and most recently web sites, tend to assume the place of academic journals. Material published here is not subject to the standards of rigorous criticism and needless to say, the result is a labyrinth of misinformation, unsubstantiated claims and exaggerated conclusions. Their defenders hide behind the 'smoke screen' that the orthodox publications are controlled by the establishment; that there is no openness to new ideas, but only a conflict of interest and bias. They resort even to the media and 'pop' press. Publications from 'Rodale' Press, the ever popular 'Prevention ' magazine and a flood of other quasi-health magazines with a range of suggestive 'health' titles, are the new popular forum for these natural health alternatives. They speak directly to the consuming public who can assert their right to know. Add to that the rising tide of 'health' books that appear from week to week and the misinformation becomes a tidal wave. But this may be defeating its own cause for in the end, only good science will remain. The best of nature as demonstrated by the best of science will survive all bias and controversy.

The Cancer Conspiracy?

Speaking of controversy, there is probably no more important controversy between the orthodox allopathic medical establishment and the dissident, alternative health-care practitioners and their supporters, than in their different approaches and conclusions with respect to cancer.

Cancer is the second leading cause of death in North America. It now kills more people in a single year than all of World Wide II did. Cancer research has been at the center stage of medicine ever since President Nixon declared 'War on Cancer' three decades ago. Some advances have been made, but after countless millions of dollars have been spent on research, cancer is still with us in epidemic proportions – at least one in three persons are now likely to get it and most of those are likely to die from it. Some are quick to point out that cancer is not only a terrible disease, but it is also a multi-billion dollar industry. There is an estimated $30 billion expenditure on cancer research in the U.S. alone. There is also an increasing volume of *alternative* literature that seeks to establish a case for an organized conspiracy on the part of the Establishment. This Establishment it is argued, includes the government, major corporations, the medical establishment, the pharmaceutical industry, medical equipment manufacturers, cancer organizations, and even much of the news media. Just a cursory look at recent popular books on the subject, commonly available in health food stores or on the Internet, makes the debate obvious.

For example, *The Cancer Conspiracy* by John J. Moelaert (1999) argues that cancer is much more of a political problem than a medical one. The so-called war against cancer is, in reality, largely 'a gigantic hoax and cruel illusion.' The main battle is between corporate wealth and public health, he contends. To understand the politics of cancer one must penetrate the mass of misinformation generated by the cancer industry. To varying degrees they all distort and often suppress critical cancer information. People are denied their fundamental rights to know the facts about cancer, thereby impairing their ability to make informed decisions. 'If all the years of cancer research had been as effective as claimed and if all the so-called medical breakthroughs had been real, obviously fewer and fewer people would get and die of cancer, instead of more and more. The reality is that the public is being misled on a massive scale.'

The year before, renowned cancer expert Dr. Samuel S. Epstein updated and revised his classic work in *'The Politics of Cancer Revisited'* which sought to explain why we are losing what should be the winnable war against cancer. It attacked the misdirected policies of the cancer establishment, particularly the National Cancer Institute and the American Cancer Society which have monopolized the government funding and the public understanding of cancer. He insisted that there is a clear conflict of interest which has led to an unbalanced fixation on damage control – diagnosis and treatment – and on molecular biology, with a "not always benign indifference to cancer prevention." In a glowing introduction, Congressman John Conyers (D., Michigan) wrote:

"This new book argues that the Cancer Establishment has become beset with a range of myopic institutional pressures which prevent it from devoting more research and capital to prevention: the common quest to amass more resources and build bigger empires by the research institutions which promise what may be a mythical pot of gold at the end of the research rainbow; the apparently growing and somewhat disturbing interlocking corporate interests of pharmaceutical industries who benefit from public optimism that an elixir is near, and chemical industries that want as little prevention through environmental regulation as possible. While political scientists commonly

theorize that all institutions may be subject to these pressures, no one has attempted to systematically document these problems in the context of the war against cancer until now.

"None of this is to say that research into the mechanisms, treatment and potential cures of cancer is not critical or that it should not continue. It should. None of this is to say that there are not noble people struggling to find cures. There are. But, THE POLITICS OF CANCER Revisited argues that as important as the research is, it cannot eclipse prevention. We should not in our emotionally understandable hope for a cure become transfixed with a Nero-like neglect for the simple truth that preventing cancer appears to be well within our grasp."

Most recently, Ron Gdanski has written *'CANCER – Cause, Cure and Cover-up'* (2000) in which he sites hundreds of sources to establish three major propositions:

1. *"We know the cause of cancer.* We know that parasitic living things in our body cause human cells to mutate cell-wall membranes during replication; either during normal growth and cell replacement, or to repair an injury. Nutritional and mineral deficiencies and toxins reduce immune system function allowing for fungal and parasitic infection. Infection leads to the substitution of microbial enzymes and proteins for human enzymes and proteins. All degenerative diseases follow this path.

2. *We know that the cure for cancer lies in removing the causes.* Cancer is caused by microbial infections.

3. *We know there is a serious cover-up in progress.* We have also reviewed several remarkable cancer cures that are suppressed, and we know why they work, because we understand the true cause of cancer. We know that the cancer epidemic is a man-made phenomenon, and controlled by authorities who are defrauding the public on a massive scale.

Gdanski draws much on the earlier publication *"The Cure For*

All Cancers" (1993) by naturopath Dr. Hulda Clark but he does find a major disagreement:

"The important thing to realize about what I consider to be an error in Dr. Clark's theory that microbial growth factors cause cells to replicate is that it doesn't really matter in regard to the cure for cancer. She claims microbial growth factors cause cells to replicate and mutate. I claim that the current of injury causes cells to replicate, and the growth factors only mutate the cell-wall membrane. Curing cancer by eliminating parasites is the same in either case."

This is the kind of stuff that is popularized among the *alternative* culture. It is not often based on science. It is more often the desperate cry from those who insist on simple answers and so turn back to nature. They want apparent results more urgently than they seek the truth. Some Cancer patients get exposed to it or listen to testimonials and then vote with their feet. They go off to Mexico, the Bahamas or elsewhere to attend *alternative* cancer clinics often staffed by good North American specialists who themselves voted with their feet and found a haven where they could practice with their best skills and knowledge for their patients' benefit. Unfortunately, their clinics have got a bad wrap in the media. Many good Case Reports have gone unnoticed and the sensational misadventures have been exploited in the media. However, there is something to learn here, it is not all bogus.

Clearly, there is some inertia in the orthodox cancer establishment and many influences have dictated the course of the 'war on cancer'. There would be much to gain now that *alternative* approaches are slowly being recognized. **If only for the patients' sake, nature and science must come to a cohesion rather than a collision, if we are ever to win the real war.**

The Natural Hypothesis

Underlying the accusations of a cancer conspiracy and much of the explanations and claims for most of the natural alternative therapies, is a fundamental, though unproven hypothesis, which keeps reappearing in all discussions on the subject. It is a presumed universal answer to most probing questions regarding mechanisms of physiological action. This general hypothesis may be summarized as follows:

I.   **The Immune System is paramount to health.**
Nature has endowed human (animal) life with a resil-
ient, self-protective defense mechanism that we call the
immune system.

II.   **The Immune System is often compromised.**
Human beings become susceptible to poor health when
nature is neglected (by omission) or abused (by com-
mission). Poor lifestyle habits (including diet and nutrition, exercise, stress management and thought patterns), drugs and toxins from the environment, are the
major factors to suppress the immune response.

III. **Sickness comes from a weakened Immune System.**
Disease (otherwise exploited as dis-ease) or sub-opti-
mal health results when extrinsic or intrinsic variables
overwhelm this depressed immune system. Symptoms
are only the manifestations of the root cause.

IV.   **Natural therapies attack the root cause by strength-
ening the Immune System.**
The mechanism and goal of any natural therapy is to
restore or strengthen the immune system to its optimal
functioning, so that the normal healthy course of nature can resume. And all this, without impacting the
normal functioning of the body as a whole.

V.   **A strong Immune System allows the body to heal
itself.**
Left alone to itself, nature is wiser than man and can
maintain health when given the right input and treated
correctly. It is therefore best to let nature take its course
whenever possible.

The tenets of this general hypothesis form the proposed rationale for many different alternative therapies. Each proponent wants to
fall back on this like a crutch to support whatever product or service
they would recommend. It appeals to the lowest common denominator.
After all, every individual does have an indispensable immune system
which does have this central protective role. That is self-evident.

But the immune system is not some vague, ethereal product of the imagination. It is a very real anatomical and physiological system with many discrete units that have specific functions. Over the past few decades, many researchers have worked diligently to understand the detailed mechanisms involved. The appearance of AIDS has increased these efforts but many other clinical challenges have driven this major research in laboratories and hospitals around the world. It has relevance for things like allergy, immunization, blood transfusion, organ transplants, prosthetic implants, auto-immunity, degenerative diseases and much, much more. The application of empirical science has unlocked the doors to make the sophisticated clinical management of these conditions possible. It has saved countless millions of lives.

Therein is the irony. Alternative practitioners and promoters talk about the immune system. They make reference to it at every turn. They make it central to their philosophy and to almost every proposed health intervention. Some question the general approach and even the competence of orthodox clinicians in dealing with anything short of acute illness and trauma. Yet the evidence is clearly on the side of allopathic doctors and scientists who have applied *the scientific method* to unravel the intricate secrets of *nature* in protecting the body against disease. Just think of the array of modern medical achievements. Immunology is still a relatively young science but we know enough now to practice a rational *science* of medicine, while wisdom still dictates that we never dispose of its *art*.

In the next chapter we will review what we do know from *science* about this all-important immune system and then we will be ready to tap into *nature's* goldmine to find a surprising contribution.

PART
2

DEFENDING
THE
BODY

Chapter Four

THE IMMUNE SYSTEM
Unraveling some Secrets of Nature

J ust a few decades ago, even doctors were receiving little instruction in Immunology because little was known. Today, this has become one of the most rapidly advancing fields of science and medicine, making an impact on the entire world. The immune system is at the heart of major health problems everywhere. From traditional infectious diseases and allergy, to the big challenges of AIDS and cancer, and the increasing opportunities of universal immunization and organ transplantation. As the research continues we are witnessing the triumph of the scientific method as secrets of nature are being exploited in the service of man.

In this chapter we want to explore some of the basic science underlying the immune system. We could never do justice to this vast area in so short a space and time, but we want to illustrate how *nature* and *science*, at their concerted best, provide new horizons for health and quality of life.

IMPORTANCE

Just imagine, your body is indeed constantly under attack from bacteria, viruses, radiation, chemicals from without and within, as well as, mutations, trauma, etc. In fact, when one reflects on the wide variety of insults to which each of us is exposed every day, it is surprising that we do not fall victim to illness and disease more frequently. No person is an island and we do not live in a controlled biosphere. On the contrary, we are surrounded by a world of hostile microorganisms that do all they can to survive at our expense, and an environment of chemicals and radiation that threatens to wipe us out, if we are not careful.

The importance of the immune system cannot be overemphasized. When all the professional health care workers have done their best, one must still be obliged to wait and see how any given person will react in the face of whatever threatening health situation they may encounter. In a sense, that is the ultimate measure of true physical fitness.

When exposed to insult or challenge, your cells fight back by a complex series of *inter-* and *intra-* cellular events, which in total, is generally referred to as the immune response. They declare war on the invading enemy. They could lose a battle, now and then, but they must win the war! In real terms therefore, your health depends on you or more precisely, on your immune system. In fact, your life depends on it!

Your immune system is a highly sophisticated and complex network of specialized cells and organs that exists to defend your body against attacks by "foreign" invaders. When it is functioning properly, it is able to fight off infections by threatening agents such as bacteria, viruses, fungi and parasites. When it malfunctions, however, it can open doorways to disease.

Severe defects in immunity are frequently incompatible with life. No person reading this could possibly have survived childhood without an intact immune system. Immuno-deficiences of T-cells give rise to fungal infections, pneumocystis pneumonia, herpes-virus and other viral infections. This is exemplified in the worst way by AIDS patients who succumb to similar opportunistic infections. Defects in antibody production tend to produce recurrent bacterial sepsis, as well as certain specific virus infections and some arthritis. Either form can lead to lymphoma or certain other tumors, probably due to unchecked effects of certain DNA viruses. These are just a few examples of what can and does happen when the immune system fails to execute effectively.

Your immune system, which could be compared in complexity to the intricacies of your brain and nervous system, displays several remarkable characteristics. It can distinguish between your "self" and "nonself". It is able to remember previous experiences and react accordingly. The system displays both enormous diversity and extraordinary specificity; not only is it able to recognize many millions of distinctive nonself molecules, it can produce molecules and cells to match up with and counteract each one of them specifically. It has at its command a sophisticated array of weapons for this cellular warfare.

The success of this system in defending your body relies on an incredibly elaborate and dynamic regulatory-communications network. Millions and millions of cells, organized into sets and subsets for specific functions, pass information back and forth like clouds of bees swarming around a hive. The result is a sensitive system of checks and balances which produces an immune response that is prompt, appropriate, effective and self-limiting. But we get caught up in the details. Let's begin the discussion by taking a panoramic view of the big picture.

THE BIG PICTURE

Your overall defense system contains both non-specific and specific elements. The non-specific defenses include the skin and mucous membranes; secretions with special characteristics like stomach acid; normal flora of commensal organisms that maintain a balanced ecology; a number of cell types that do general labor and clean up (typically white cells); and a few components that carry out very important work but only on command, such as the complement system. The highly specific immune system is reserved for B- and T- lymphocytes which we will discuss in some detail later.

The principal components of the complete protection system, identified here in anatomical structure and functional terms for convenience, are summarized in Table 3. Following are some key characteristics and what you can do about them.

THE SKIN.   The skin is the largest organ in your body. It performs many crucial functions including being an effective barrier to environmental threats, both physical and biological. When anyone suffers from severe burns for example, there is a medical crisis due to the extreme challenges to the body's defenses. **KEY**: *To avoid dehydration and infection. Avoid sun damage. Treat burns.*
THE RESPIRATORY TRACT. Special linings in the airways, including the nasal passages and throat, protect your lungs from foreign particulate matter and also from smoke and chemical inhalation. The

TABLE 3.   OVERVIEW OF YOUR BODY'S PROTECTION

STRUCTURE		FUNCTION
EXTERNAL		
THE SKIN	⇨	Barrier
EPITHELIAL LININGS		
• Respiratory Tract	⇨	Breathing
• Gastrointestinal Tract	⇨	Eating
• Urogenital Tract	⇨	Intimacy
• Auditory Canal	⇨	Hearing
INTERNAL		
ORGANS		
• Liver	⇨	Pollution Plant
• ·Kidneys	⇨	Filtration
• Lymph Nodes & Spleen	⇨	Processing
• Bone Marrow	⇨	Production
• Thymus Gland	⇨	Maturation
CELLS		
• The Immune System	⇨	Defense Force
MOLECULES		
• Antibodies	⇨	Weapons
• Cytokines	⇨	Triggers
• Antioxidants	⇨	Stabilizers

latter usually triggers coughing to facilitate expulsion. **KEY**: *Avoid polluted air and cigarette smoke.*

THE GASTRO-INTESTINAL TRACT. The daily intake of food and water passes through almost forty feet of complex tubing during which digestion and absorption are critically controlled. Vomiting and diarrhea are protective mechanisms of emptying the bowel. Chemical secretions and special linings defend against harmful contents which remain. **KEY**: *To exclude ingested poisons and metabolites. Eat healthy foods ...*

THE LIVER. The central processing of waste that gets into (or is formed in) body tissues, takes place in the liver. Many complex enzyme systems there, convert harmful products into harmless waste that is secreted into the blood stream and cleared through the kidneys or the biliary tree (gall bladder and bile). Advanced liver failure allows toxic products to get to the brain and usually leads to a medical emergency. **KEY**: *To avoid addictions, additives and abuse.*

THE BONE MARROW. The bone marrow is a very productive organ. All blood cell lines are produced in the bone marrow, including the cells of the immune system. Today, bone marrow transplantation is being used in life-saving procedures to restore blood cell production in certain clinical states. **KEY**: *A healthy, complete diet. Moderate exercise.*

THE LYMPH NODES. Almost everyone at some time has experienced swollen lymph glands or nodes. These are usually indicative of infection, or sometimes reactive inflammation and even cancer. They represent small factories for immune cells and their defensive activities. Some cells produce antibodies that are effective circulating weapons which trigger a cascade of chemical and biological warfare. Hopefully, the immune system wins. **KEY**: *Monitor and report.*

RESPONSES

In the most general terms, nearly all insults to your body in both health and disease, will result in two major consequences: First, there is a general physiological response from your organs, acting in concert to discern different priorities and re-distribute the bodies resources. Then there is the local response which gets right down to defense at the microscopic level.

1. The GENERAL Immune Response

The first major consequence when your body is threatened is a common pattern of retaliation, by which you prepare 'for fight or flight.' Most of this happens spontaneously by reflex action, often before or even without your conscious thought. It was broadly identified as the Stress Adaptation Syndrome.

*At the **MACRO** level: The major physiological systems adapt under varying conditions to maximize your chances of survival and safeguard your health. For example, you can experience your heart racing, fever, exposed blood clotting, changes in urinary output, circulation, gut motility, muscle tone... etc.*

The net effect is to maintain or restore what is called the state of 'homeostasis' in which the healthy body thrives. It was the famous nineteenth century French physiologist, Claude Bernard, who first observed that *"the constancy of the internal environment (i.e. homeostasis) is the condition for a free life"*.

Life is maintained then in a healthy state only within very narrow ranges of all the physiological variables. Feedback and reflex control mechanisms allow the body to adapt quickly and effectively when challenged. Survival itself may be at stake but at least, our state of health is critically determined by this adaptation capacity. This is the most important sign of robust or dynamic health.

2. The LOCAL Immune Response

As was noted before, the second major consequence arising from any insult to your body is targeted at the local level. It may take different forms, but the overall strategy may be classified broadly into an inflammatory response and an immune response.

The *inflammatory* response is somewhat more pathological but essentially, it is a process consisting of a dynamic complex of reactions that occur in the affected blood vessels and related tissues, in response to any injury or abnormal stimulation caused by some physical, chemical or biological agent. The classical cardinal signs are *rubor* (redness), *calor* (heat), *tumor* (swelling) and *dolor* (pain). Function can also be affected. These common inflammatory changes are usually gross enough to be observed. They occur at the tissue level even though they are triggered by complex cellular activity.

The *immune* response on the other hand , is generally invisible though no less significant. As we have said, it is cellular warfare. The cell is under attack and it is prepared to fight back.

*At the **MICRO** level: Each cell is a living entity that has unique characteristics of 'homeostasis' too, even in the microbiological world. The cell exploits molecular biology and genetics to first protect itself. Then the specific cells of the immune system are able to participate in an orchestrated collective response that is differentiated and very specific. This spontaneous retaliation is most effective in defense of organic life and is subject to regulatory control.*

There are three major challenges that confront **all** your cells *internally*:
- Free radicals ('hot' fragments)
- Oxidation   (oxygenated products)
- Xenobiotics (poisons)

Free Radicals. Chemical bonds between atoms typically involve the sharing of paired electrons. This leads to stable covalent molecules. When a chemical bond is broken by some reaction or another, the fragments produced each have 'unpaired' electrons which make them most unstable and therefore highly reactive. They become chemically 'hot' and attack other susceptible molecules. These may include critical nucleic acids or proteins and when DNA or RNA is involved, genetic control of cellular activity is compromised. ***Free Radicals must therefore be quenched before they destroy cells and damage tissues.***

Oxidation. Most important chemical reactions inside cells often (in fact, usually) involve oxygen or other red-ox (reduction – oxidation) systems. The simple transfer of an electron or proton from one atom to another has major consequences. Oxygen is the ubiquitous key and must be controlled. When premature oxidation takes place in cells (with superoxide-, hydroxyl- and peroxy- radicals as the lethal intermediates) these cells can be devastated. ***Such toxic intermediates must be***

neutralized before they cause a cascade to cell death.

Xenobiotics.   Poisonous chemicals can be inhaled or ingested and they eventually would end up in the circulation and body tissues. Other products of digestion and metabolism can also become toxic to cells. *All these must be neutralized before they cause damage.*
    The toxic metabolites formed inside the cell are best neutralized on-site inside the cell. Other xenobiotics can be transported to the liver to be neutralized and transformed into more harmless products and later excreted via the kidneys and biliary tract.

CHALLENGES

    As we have just seen, at the most fundamental level, cells must protect themselves individually from their own malfunction and destruction. They must neutralize and eliminate those toxic free-radicals, oxygenated species and xenobiotics to remain healthy and vigorous. That too is a level of immunity that even doctors do not commonly think about. These healthy cells can then become the units of defense in an overall strategy of protection, which opposes any invader from without or rebel from within that threatens the body as a whole. This second level is the usual level of the immune system that we think about. It is the focus of clinical training and practice. But Fig. 2 shows the different conceptual levels of defense at which the total immune system functions. This is schematic but it is also real. Only healthy cells can mount a systemic immune response, which in turn protects all the organs of the body and in effect, the total body. At this second level, where circulating cells act specifically and in concert to destroy the enemy, the immune system has at least four broad challenges to reckon with.

(i)   *To identify the enemy.* At the heart of the immune system is the ability to distinguish between 'self' and 'non-self'. The system must be able to distinguish what is friend or foe, for you or against you. Virtually every cell in each body carries distinctive surface markers (molecules) that identify it as 'self.' It is the basic identification card, or more like a uniform on the outside, for the trillions of cells that coexist peaceably in a state known as self-tolerance. But when the immune

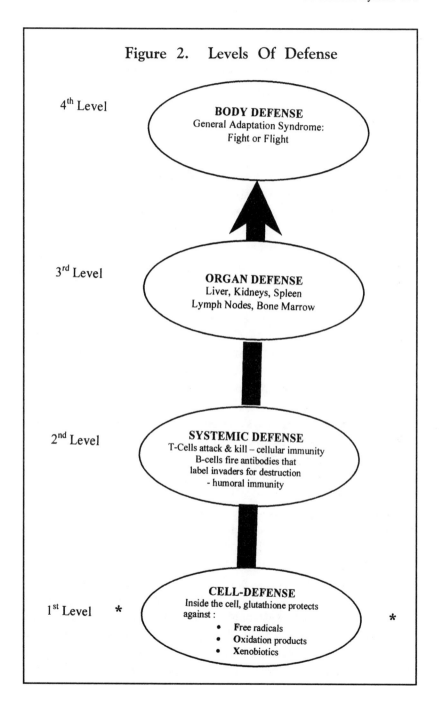

Figure 2.   Levels Of Defense

4th Level

BODY DEFENSE
General Adaptation Syndrome:
Fight or Flight

3rd Level

ORGAN DEFENSE
Liver, Kidneys, Spleen
Lymph Nodes, Bone Marrow

2nd Level

SYSTEMIC DEFENSE
T-Cells attack & kill – cellular immunity
B-cells fire antibodies that
label invaders for destruction
- humoral immunity

1st Level   *

CELL-DEFENSE
Inside the cell, glutathione protects
against :
- Free radicals
- Oxidation products
- Xenobiotics

*

defenders encounter different cells, proteins or organisms carrying surface markers or molecules that say "foreign", the immune troops move quickly to eliminate the intruders. To survive, everything in the system must wear 'the same badge' or else…!

(ii)   *To carry out immuno-surveillance.* There are millions of different possible invaders of healthy bodies. In order to accommodate enough cells to oppose any possible intruder, the immune system stores a relatively small number of each specificity in its arsenal. But when any threat appears, those few specifically matched cells are stimulated on cue, to multiply into a full- scale army. It is important that the response be specific. The system must also be on constant alert so that its defense is quick and overwhelming, before the enemy strikes a serious blow.

(iii)   *To fight back.* When activated, immune system lymphocytes must respond. They multiply and become effector cells that essentially do one or more of three things: (1) secrete lymphokines that affect other cells (spread the declaration of war); (2) kill targets bearing the activating antigen (face the enemy in direct combat and go for the kill); (3) secrete antibodies that react with the antigen (pin down the enemy and prepare them for swift and certain destruction). Each cell has a defined role and the whole operation is orchestrated with checks and balances to guarantee maximum efficiency. The immune system must be effective and complete in devastating the challenge from any perceived enemy. This is war and not a cellular picnic.

(iv)   *To turn-off or shut-down when it has done its job.* The immune response is truly one of defense. It must never be overzealous so as to be offensive against the body itself. In abnormal situations, the immune system can wrongly identify self as non-self and execute a misdirected immune attack. The result can then be an autoimmune condition or disease. In other circumstances, an apparently harmless substance can provoke the system to set off an inappropriate and harmful response which we know as an allergy. In the worst case scenario, cells of the immune system can proliferate uncontrollably; the result is cancer. For example, leukemias are caused by the proliferation of white

blood cells or leukocytes. The uncontrolled growth of antibody producing (plasma) cells can lead to multiple myeloma. Cancers of the lymphoid organs, known as lymphomas, include Hodgkin's disease.

All these challenges must be met successfully and simultaneously. To that end, the immune system has a highly sophisticated repertoire of specialized cells which execute their varied functions in a highly coordinated manner. The system stockpiles a tremendous arsenal of cells as forces and weapons. Some staff the general defenses, while others are trained on highly specific targets. To work effectively however, most immune cells require the active cooperation of their partners. Sometimes they communicate through direct physical contact, and at other times, by releasing versatile chemical messengers.

The entire system is internally regulated by genetic coding of the differentiated cell lines. Only the cells of the immune system are sufficient for the task. The application of *science* through any clinical intervention, only seeks at best, to exploit what *nature* does efficiently and consistently by cellular design. At the same time, any claim for a *natural* product or therapeutic technique to enhance the immune system must related in some way to the *science* that we now know about this sophisticated operation. We do know a lot more about its responses, including how the defense force is deployed.

YOUR DEFENSE FORCE

Every discipline has its own vocabulary and concepts. The immune system is no different. Let's define some key elements of the immune battlefield where one's health is often won or lost.

ANTIGEN.   This refers to any substance (usually a macromolecule) which, on being recognized by the immune system as **foreign**, can bind to an immune cell receptor and stimulate an immune response. That response is specific. If the binding is strong and other conditions for stimulation are fulfilled, antigen triggers the receptor-bearing cell and a response of proliferation and differentiation follows. The clone expands and acquires new functions.

ANTIBODY. This is one of a wide variety of secreted proteins elicited in an animal by different antigens. They react specifically with each particular antigen to **trigger** a variety of outcomes. They can slow down and kill viruses and bacteria.

PRIMARY RESPONSE. This is the formation of antibody after **first exposure** to an antigen. When the clone of lymphocytes which has been stimulated by its specific antigen is no longer exposed to antigen, it goes into a resting state. It retains a memory of the fact that it has been stimulated and is poised for a repeat challenge.

SECONDARY RESPONSE. This is the formation of antibody after a **second exposure** to the same antigen. It is an accelerated response (that is, faster) and an exaggerated response (that is, of much greater magnitude). Memory and the secondary response explain how one exposure to a foreign microbe (for example, a chicken pox virus) can produce life long resistance specific to that organism. It is the basis of immunization procedures.

The specificity of the primary and secondary responses is very high and cannot be overemphasized. Each particular antigen binds to only a minority of the clones of lymphocytes present and does not affect the others. **The body's defense therefore is not general, it is not some vague overall response to threat of injury or disease. It is most specific and targeted at the molecular level.**

Distinguishing Cells. Until comparatively recently, white blood cells could be distinguished only microscopically by size or the ability to take up certain dyes with different patterns. Those techniques, however, were not helpful for discrimination between different populations of lymphocytes, since the smaller lymphocytes are almost indistinguishable by light microscopy. A major breakthrough came about when different reagents or defining markers were found to react with the surface of different cells. For example, the surface of the human T-cell was found to react with sheep red blood cells to form characteristic "rosettes". As this reaction was found to be quite specific, it provided a convenient way to purify human T-cells from other blood cells.

There are a large number of different proteins on the surface of cells. The development of monoclonal antibodies gave an enormous impetus to the mapping of cell surface molecules. They allow for both the purification and characterization of cells. The cell-surface markers are now uniformly classified by the acronym CD (Cluster of Differentiation) followed by a number indicating the sequence of their acceptance. Over 130 such cell-surface molecules have been identified. It is presumed that every protein expressed in the cell surface has some natural ligand that binds to it, and thus the surface-expressed molecule plays some role in receiving a signal from outside the cell and transmitting that information into the cell.

The lymphocyte is the key cell in the immune system. The body has about one trillion of these lymphocytes which are of two major varieties. T-cells and B-cells.

T – CELLS. A variety of lymphocytes originate in the bone marrow and are processed by the **Thymus gland**. They have *specific receptors* on their surface, which have been well characterized in terms of molecular biology.

Each T-cell receptor is a unique complex of two non-identical protein chains which are bonded together by disulfide bonds. One terminal of each chain is embedded in the cell membrane and sticks into the cell's cytoplasm. The major part of each chain lives outside the cell where it can bind to complementary structures. Each one is coded for by unique rearrangements of the antibody cell receptor genes.

A typical gene consists of a fixed segment of DNA, which directs the manufacture of a given protein molecule (eg. insulin). Antibody genes, in contrast, are assembled from bits and pieces of DNA scattered widely throughout the genetic materials. As the T-cell matures, it rearranges or shuffles these gene components, picking and choosing among hundreds of DNA segments. Intervening segments of DNA are cut out; the selected pieces are spliced together. The new gene and the new T-cell receptor it now encodes are virtually unique. T-cell receptor genes do not mutate as they proliferate.

In general, T-cells do not produce circulatory antibody. Those of one type have effector or regulator functions, while another type are so-called "killer cells." The T-cell effector functions are of two varieties. *Specific* cytotoxicity refers to the direct destruction of other cells bearing the specific antigen to which the T-cells are sensitized. This is therefore known as cellular immunity. Delayed-type-hypersensitivity on the other hand, involves the organization of *non-specific* inflammation by the release of lymphokines, which are soluble proteins by which T-cells influence other cells. Similarly, the T-cell regulator functions are of two types: T-helper cells advance the war, while T-suppressor cells seek to end the conflict when the decisive battle is over. They declare the truce.

B – CELLS. These lymphocytes are mainly generated in the **Bone marrow**. They are defined by the expression of immunoglobulins on their surface which form specific receptors. When a B-cell meets antigen, under the right conditions, the antigen binds to and triggers the B-cell. When stimulated (and only then), the B-cells can proliferate (to form clones), mature into plasma cells and secrete specific antibody. This is a type of specialized **chemical warfare**. Antibodies circulate in body fluids to find specific antigens and trigger other immune responses. Usually, that means death to the enemy! This is known as humoral immunity.

Each immunoglobulin molecule (Ig, receptor or antibody) consists of two light protein chains and two heavy chains. These chains all fall into different classes, and so do the resulting immunoglobulins (IgG, M, A, D, E). For example, the IgG molecule is the commonest class of circulating antibody and consists of two so-called gamma heavy chains and two lambda light chains. IgG is able to enter tissue spaces; it works efficiently to coat microorganisms, speeding their uptake by other cells in the immune system. IgM, which usually combines in star-shaped clusters, tends to remain in the bloodstream, where it is very effective in killing bacteria. IgA concentrates in body fluids-tears, saliva, the secretions of the respiratory and gastrointestinal tracts-guarding the entrances to the body. IgE, which under normal circumstances occurs only in trace amounts, probably evolved as a defense against parasites, but it is more familiar as the villain in allergic reactions. IgD is almost exclusively found inserted into the membranes of B cells, where it somehow regulates the cell's activation. Each immunoglobulin is coded for by a unique rearrangement of specific Ig genes.

The function of the B-cell is to make antibody. This antibody binds to antigen, and can produce several outcomes. Some large antigens (eg. a malarial parasite) may be unaffected by antibody binding to its surface. There may be a direct effect of clumping (agglutination of particles or precipitation of soluble molecules); neutralization of the effects of antigen such as toxins; or occasionally, triggering of antigen-bearing cells. Binding could activate a system of proteins called complement which is lethal in defense. This complement system is made up of a series of about 25 proteins that work to "complement" the activity of antibodies in destroying bacteria, either by facilitating phagocytosis or by puncturing the bacterial cell membrane. Complement proteins circulate in the blood in an inactive form. When the first of the complement substances is triggered, it sets in motion a ripple effect. As each component is activated in turn, it acts upon the next in a precise sequence of carefully regulated steps known as the "complement cascade." It drives the classic inflammatory response, ties up the invading enemy and then unleashes a barrage of strikes that cause bacteriolysis and cell death. In a word, antibody combines with antigen to ignite the troops, intensify the battle and accelerate victory for the home forces. They may be eventually removed from the circulation by clearing mechanisms in the liver and the spleen.

Both T - Cell and B - Cell lymphocytes are stimulated when their specific receptors combine with foreign material of complementary structure and undergo clonal expansion by the millions. That is a unique characteristic of the immune system. It distinguishes a T-cell lymphocyte, say, from other white blood cells like polymorphonuclear leukocytes, which do not have any clone-specific receptors that differ from one another. The uniqueness of each clone of lymphocytes resides in the unique amino acid sequence of its receptor, as determined by a unique rearrangement of the receptor genes in each clone.

ANTIGEN PRESENTING CELLS.   T-cell receptors do not bind soluble native antigen very well. They bind to the antigen which has been degraded or processed by the antigen-presenting cells. There are several morphologically distinct classes of cells which process such antigens non-specifically and prepare them for **presentation** to the T-helper cells like military **ESCORTS**. They serve like front-line agents making arrests and bringing the culprits to swift and certain justice.

Further to this, when T-cells see any specific antigen or antigen-presenting cells, they must see it in association with a set of proteins called the major histocompatibility (MHC) complex. MHC products fall into two general classes, I and II, and then several sub-categories. An MHC probably exists in all mammals but in the case of humans in particular, the MHC is known as the HLA complex. These protein products serve as critical identifying labels and are used to "type" individuals for compatibility especially with respect to organ and bone marrow transplantation. But the real function of the MHC is immunoregulatory and it is only related to transplantation per se by coincidence. Its products are essential antigen-presenting structures in the reactions of T-cells with specific antigens. Some specific MHC labels are associated with specific disease incidences such as ankylosing spondylitis, multiple sclerosis or juvenile-onset diabetes.

T – HELPER CELLS. They are the small T-lymphocytes that act as the **COMMANDERS-IN-CHIEF** of the immune system. They have that regulatory function. They recognize processed antigen, become activated, and in turn, trigger responses from other members of the defense force. They therefore exert a positive effect on the growth or differentiation of other lymphocytes, including either T-cells or B-cells. The effect is mediated by the same soluble factors that we call lymphokines. These potent and diverse chemical messengers include the clinically important interleukin-2, gamma-interferon, and many others. They can encourage cell growth, promote cell activation, direct cellular traffic, destroy some target cells and incite macrophages. They are distinguished by CD4 markers and look for antigen bound to a Class II MHC molecule – a combination displayed by macrophages and B-cells.

Actually, CD4 is just one of a number of membrane proteins on T-cells. These include CD3, CD4 and CD8. CD3 is intimately associated with the T-cell receptor on all T-cells. It is a complex of three polypeptides and maybe a switch for activating the T-cell after its specific receptor binds antigen. On the other hand, CD4 and CD8 are mutually exclusive membrane proteins, each occurring on one subset of lymphocytes. CD4 is the particular set of membrane proteins on the T-helper subset of T-cells and they are also present on the T-cells involved with the delayed-type hypersensitivity reactions. CD8 is the different membrane protein on a subset of T-cells with predominately cytotoxic and suppressor functions. The CD4+ and CD8+ subsets each interact preferentially with one class of MHC antigen-presenting products (CD4 with Class II and CD8 with Class I respectively).

CD3, CD4 and CD8 are widely used as markers in clinical medicine.

T – KILLER CELLS. These **PARATROOPERS** activated by the T-helper cells have only one goal: to destroy the enemy before it has time to multiply. They wipe-out virus-infected cells and perform immune surveillance. They are distinguished by CD8 markers and look for antigen bound to a Class I MHC molecule which are found on almost all body cells.

K – CELLS. These are the immune **THUGS**. They are subpopulations of non-B, non-T mononuclear cells and are responsible for lysis (destruction) of cells with antigen - antibody complexes.

NK – CELLS. These are medium sized lymphocytes more like **HIRED THUGS**. They also have no B-cell or T-cell markers but possess characteristic granules. Like cytotoxic T-cells, these granules contain potent chemicals. They can, without specific recognition, spontaneously kill-off transformed (cancerous) cells or virally infected cells. They kill on contact. The killer binds to its target, aims its weapons and then delivers a lethal burst of chemicals that produce holes in the target cell's membrane. Fluids seep in and leak out, and the cell bursts. It's a merciless onslaught. In several immunodeficiency diseases, including AIDS, natural killer cell function is abnormal.

The immune response is carefully orchestrated. Each type of cell is genetically programmed and equipped for its specialized tasks.

MACROPHAGES. They are the **GROUND FORCES** that roam throughout the body, consuming pollutants and other invaders at a restless rate. Their activity can be enhanced by antigen-specific T-cells which release soluble products. When activated in this manner, macrophages can distinguish between normal and transformed cells.

Macrophages represent one type of large white cells called phagocytes (literally "cell eaters" or scavengers) that can engulf and digest marauding microorganisms and other antigenic particles. Some phagocytes also have the ability to present antigen to lymphocytes. The more important phagocytes include *monocytes* and macrophages. Monocytes themselves circulate in the blood, then migrate into tissues where they develop into macrophages ("big eaters"). Like efficient ground troops, macrophages are seeded and camouflaged throughout body tissues in a variety of guises. They are versatile cells that play many roles. They specialize in mop-up operations. As scavengers, they rid the body of worn-out cells and other debris. Foremost among the cells that "present" antigen to T cells, having first digested and processed it, macrophages play a crucial role in initiating the immune response. As secretory cells, monocytes and macrophages are vital to the regulation of immune responses and the development of inflammation; they churn out an amazing array of powerful chemical substances (monokines) including enzymes, complement proteins, and regulatory factors such as interleukin-1. At the same time, they carry receptors for lymphokines that allow them to be "activated" into single-minded pursuit of microbes and tumor cells.

MAST CELLS. These are the **WEATHERMEN**. Large cells (and their precursor, basophils) bind specifically with a class of immunoglobulins which then combine with antigens in bridge-pairs resulting in release of vasoactive amines, particularly **histamine**. This histamine release is responsible for the clinical allergy reactions. They do not circulate like basophils but remain stationed on guard in the lungs, skin, tongue, and linings of the nose and intestinal tract. They have a dedicated job to do, and they execute it well.

T – SUPPRESSOR CELLS. These are the other group of T-cells with regulator functions (opposite to T-helper cells). They are the **FLAG-**

BEARERS. Small lymphocytes, they will call off the battle when victory has been   achieved. They tell T-KILLER cells to stop the fight. They also carry the CD8 marker.

T – MEMORY CELLS. These cells stay in the body after the primary exposure or infection. They are **DATA-PROCESSORS** trained to recognize the invasion of the same enemy in the future.

B – MEMORY CELLS. They function in the same way as T-memory cells. They will produce antibodies in the secondary response, upon recognizing the same enemy. They initiate rapid, exaggerated response like **MARINES**. That's the basis for immunization vaccines.

The Immune Response is usually protective but if the system fails to be discriminating, civil war erupts. The body can then treat particular normal cells or parts as the enemy – that's the basis of many auto-immune diseases.

HYPERSENSITIVITY

Clinically, infections and other tissue injury manifest themselves, you will recall, through the five classic symptoms of the inflammatory response-redness, warmth, swelling, pain, and loss of function. Redness and warmth develop when, under the influence of lymphokines and complement components, small blood vessels in the vicinity of the infection become dilated and carry more blood. Swelling results when the vessels, made leaky by yet other immune secretions, allow fluid and soluble immune substances to seep into the surrounding tissue, and immune cells to converge on the site.

Many immune reactions themselves can produce tissue injury. They activate non-specific mechanisms which can hurt by-stander cells. More than that, sometimes the host must adopt a "scorched earth" strategy to control an aggressive invader, destroying normal tissue in the process. Sometimes an intracellular parasite such as a virus, can only be controlled by destroying the infected cell. In these and other circumstances, the immune response can produce tissue injury, a process known as hypersensitivity. These reactions fall into different broad categories.

In the first type of hypersensitivity reactions, antigen binds to IgE immunoglobulins on mast cells, releasing the highly potent mediators such as histamine and leukotrienes in their granules. This is the type of hypersensitivity seen in the mild, classical hay-fever symptoms as well as the unusual but severe anaphylactic reactions to stings, drugs or foods.

A second type of hypersensitivity was referred to earlier and is that mediated by the binding of antibody to antigen on a cell or basement membrane. This activates the lethal complement system, attracts white blood cells, and thus directly damages the antigen-bearing structure. This is the so-called Arthus reaction which is illustrated in clinical practice by autoimmune destruction of red blood cells leading to anemia, or by damage to the basement membranes of the filtering units in the kidneys.

Yet another type of hypersensitivity reaction is caused by deposition of similar antigen-antibody complexes formed in the circulation. They can precipitate out in various roles such as in the kidney, or fix complement or cause disease directly.

The final type of hypersensitivity reaction gives rise to the common delayed-type hypersensitivity phenomenon. It is a T-cell mediated inflammation. Activated T-cells can induce non-specific cells such as macrophages, to be trapped in tissue, and activated release may pharmacologically activate materials as in the very common skin test for tuberculosis. Alternatively, activated T-cells may be directly cytotoxic and kill of the enemy on direct confrontation.

Defense Summary

It is most likely that the immune system has developed as a means of ridding the body of potentially harmful foreign substances. There is no doubt that microorganisms and their products form some of the greatest dangers from which the body has to protect itself throughout life. Immunity against infection with microorganisms and against damage caused by their metabolic by-products results from a fine interaction of specific humoral and cell-mediated immune mechanisms and those cells which have the power of ingesting and digesting foreign material. The action of these cells depends on their ability to ingest foreign material by a process of phagocytosis. These cells also contain a number of granules which release a wide range of enzymes capable of digesting proteins and other large molecules that the cell has ingested. It is likely that the recognition of 'foreigness' by these cells is dependent to some degree on the interaction of humoral and cell-mediated immunity. It is possible that these cells are also able to function within the body independent of immunity. However, the presence of immunologic amplification mechanisms greatly facilitates the capacity of these cells to deal with microorganisms.

Speaking of immunity, this now leads us to discuss active immunization as the first of several major applications to which the understanding of the immune system has been put.

SCIENCE ANSWERS NATURE'S CALL

IMMUNIZATION.   Whenever T cells and B cells are activated, some of the cells become "memory" cells. Then, the next time that an individual encounters that same antigen, the immune system is primed to destroy it quickly.   "Active immunity" refers to the body mounting its own immune response and it can be triggered by both infection and vaccination. Vaccines contain microorganisms that have been altered so they will produce such an immune response, but will not be able to induce full-blown disease.

The net results of widespread immunization programs have demonstrated effective protection against infectious disease which represents an immense, if not the greatest accomplishment of biomedical science. Millions of lives have been saved and untold suffering avoided. For example, smallpox has been eradicated, poliomyelitis caused by wild-type viruses has been virtually eliminated, and measles and haemophilus influenza type b (Hib) invasive disease among children below five years of age have been reduced to record low numbers of cases. Dramatic declines in morbidity have been reported for all nine vaccine-preventable diseases for which vaccination was universally recommended for use in children before 1990. The more than one million cases in total have decreased to less than one percent. However, the viruses and bacteria that cause vaccine-preventable disease and death still exist and can be passed on to people who are not protected by vaccines.

Despite the astounding achievements of immunization practices and the advances in the science of immunology, there remains a growing number of *natural* antagonists and skeptics. There is much misinformation in some quarters where advocates of 'pop-science', in the name of nature, health and wellness, continue to spread ridiculous conclusions about the net value of immunization. They take comfort for example, in the critique of the prominent Illinois physician Dr. Robert Mendelsohn who published *Confessions of a Medical Heretic* (a bestseller of 1979) in which he questioned the relevance, safety and efficacy of some contemporary immunization protocols. We need not debate the issue here. Science must triumph. The facts must speak for themselves. Rather than being contrary to nature, immunization exploits the best of nature's defenses to protect the body against the ravages of infectious disease. The risk of any vaccine must always be taken into consideration with the risks of contracting the actual disease. Contra-indications must always be recognized. To illustrate, as recently as October 1999, the Advisory Committee on Immunization Practices voted to no longer recommend rotavirus vaccine for infants. The action was based on the results of a review of the scientific data. It showed a strong association between Rotaschield vaccine and a rare occurrence of bowel twisting or obstruction among some infants during the first 1-2 weeks following vaccination. That is the scientific method. But on balance, **the case for widespread but controlled immunization is abundantly clear. There is no substitute in nature. We know enough about the science and we have the technology to practice true disease prevention; anything less would be most irresponsible.**

BLOOD TYPING AND TRANSFUSION. The scientific discovery of the natural ABO blood group antigens established the immunologic basis for transfusion reactions. This discovery, and the subsequent discovery of the Rh antigens and the tests that were developed to determine the blood group antigens, made the life-saving transfusing of blood a practical and useful clinical procedure. Probably someone you know has had the benefit of this intervention. Most blood transfusions proceed without any significant immunologic risk because *science* has identified the major red blood cell antigens that differ between individuals of the same species, the problems they can cause, how they are detected, and how to manage patients at risk.

Thanks to good *science*, an Rh-negative woman (who has not already formed anti-Rh) who gets pregnant with an Rh-positive fetus, can be protected in almost all cases, by an intramuscular injection of Rh Immune Globulin, or when given within three days after delivery. Passively administered anti-D suppresses the antibody response to the D-positive fetal cells and provides protection against hemolytic disease in the next pregnancy.

Common blood transfusion for all patients requires careful preparation and blood typing to avoid severe transfusion reactions. Routinely the red cells of the donor and recipient are tested for the presence of the clinically most important antigens. These are the A and B of the ABO system and the D of the Rh system. Other blood group antigens are less immunogenic and, in choosing donor blood, it is not practical to take them routinely into consideration.

Transfusion may also be in principle, otherwise contaminated in a poorly screened blood supply. In particular, we have observed misadventures in recent years involving transmission of either HIV (human immunodeficiency virus) or hepatitis C virus. By the application of the scientific method, it is now common practice to screen blood donors and the blood supply per se to deliver a safe, reliable and confirmed product to patients requiring transfusions. Those with religious objections, such as Jehovah Witnesses, may in good conscience refuse blood transfusion even when medically indicated. But there is little excuse today, **with the extreme checks and balances in the blood supply, to deny proper clinical management, including blood transfusions when clearly indicated, either in the name of *nature, wellness* or any other pretext of alternative, complementary or holistic medicine.**

TRANSPLANTATION. Today, thousands of people in North America who have had serious medical problems have experienced a modern miracle of transplantation and have been able to return to active, productive lives. In the last few decades, important medical breakthroughs such as tissue typing and the development of immuno suppressive drugs have allowed for more successful organ transplants and a longer survival rate for transplant recipients. Transplants of kidneys, livers, hearts, lungs, pancreases and small bowels are now considered an accepted part of medical treatment. In addition, bone marrow transplants are saving lives and corneal transplants are restoring sight. All this is already possible through *science* and the field is still in its infancy.

But the need for organ transplants continues to exceed organ supply. It is estimated that every day, ten people on waiting lists die due to lack of transplantable organs. Every 27 minutes someone receives a new organ. More living donors are becoming available and committed and the field is accelerating. Organ transplantation has become a widespread remedy for life-threatening disease. The major bottleneck remains the availability of suitable donors and the main challenge is to minimize the threat of tissue rejection. The pursuit of that goal goes back to fundamentals of the immune system.

We now understand fairly well that the success of any transplant - whether it is accepted or rejected - depends on the stubbornness of the immune system. **For a transplanted organ to be accepted, the body of the recipient must be made to suppress its natural tendency to get rid of all foreign tissue.** That represents a major problem.

Scientists have tackled this problem in two ways. The first has been to make sure that the tissue of the donor and the recipient are as similar as possible. That calls for tissue typing, or histocompatibility testing, which involves matching the same molecular markers of self on body tissues that we discussed earlier. These are the same MHC products, and because the typing is usually done on white blood cells, or leukocytes, the markers are referred to as human leukocyte antigens (HLA). Tissue typing relies on antibodies to determine if a potential organ donor and recipient share two or more HLA antigens as determined by their respective genes, and thus are likely to make a good "match". The other approach to taming transplant rejection is to suppress the recipient's immune system. This can be achieved through a variety of powerful immunosuppressive drugs.

Not surprisingly, any such all-out assault on the immune system leaves a transplant recipient susceptible to both opportunistic infections and lymphomas. Although those patients need careful medical follow up, many of them are able to lead active and essentially normal lives.

An important consequence of attacking the immune system is the depletion of active lymphocytes and a drain on the bone marrow reservoir where the vast majority, if not all of them, originate. In fact, when the immune response is severely depressed for any reason – as the result of inherited defects, cancer therapy, or AIDS-one possible remedy is a transfer of healthy bone marrow to replenish lymphocytes and other depleted cell lines. Bone marrow transplants are also used to treat patients with cancers of the blood, the blood-forming organs, and the lymphoid system. Once in the circulation, transplanted bone marrow cells travel to the bones where the immature cells mature into functioning B-cells and T-cells.

Like other transplanted tissue, however, bone marrow from a donor must carry identity markers that closely match those of the person intended to receive it. For cancer patients who face immunosuppressive therapy but who have no readily matched donor, doctors have used "autologous" transplants: in such cases, the person's bone marrow is removed, frozen, and stored until therapy is complete; then the cells are thawed and reinfused.   What a powerful combination of *science* and *nature*!

CANCER.   The immune system provides one of the body's main defenses against cancer. We now know that when normal cells turn into cancer cells, some of the antigens on their surface change. The existence of an immune response against a tumor is based on the changes in these surface components of the malignant cells that do not occur in normal cells, and that gives rise to structures that are antigenic. These new or altered antigens flag immune defenders, including cytotoxic T-cells, natural killer cells, and macrophages. This is the same classic response to enemy attack where the cancer cells are now the enemy within, an apparent mutiny of forces in rebellion against orchestrated control.

According to one theory, patrolling cells of the immune system provide continuing bodywide surveillance, spying out and eliminating cells that undergo malignant transformation. The model sounded good, seemed to make a lot of sense and it was consistent by and large with observation. However, with further *scientific research,* the accumulating evidence has suggested more strongly that the immune system actually attacks only tumors caused by viral infections. This would account for only a minority of all cases.

Blood tests show that people can develop antibodies to many types of tumor antigens (although the antibodies may not actually be effective in fighting the tumor). Skin testing (similar to skin testing for tuberculosis) has demonstrated that tumors provoke cellular immunity as well. Furthermore, studies indicated that cancer patients have a better prognosis when their tumors are infiltrated with immune cells. Immune responses may indeed underlie the observed spontaneous disappearance of some cancers.

During the past century, excitement has waxed and waned over the possibility that this extraordinary disease-fighting prowess of the immune system might be enlisted to destroy cancers. Today doubts have vanished, and countless investigators are working to translate that same notion into potent new biological therapies.

The problem with the early primitive approach to cancer therapy was that it was nonspecific: it strengthened the overall activity of the immune system instead of selectively arousing those elements that are most able to combat cancers. During the past decade, other nonspecific immunotherapies have been developed. Needless to say, it is common for the alternative medicine advocates and proponents of all kinds of *natural* remedies to resort to the same vague generalization for their unsubstantiated claims. They often insist that their cancer remedy boosts the body's immune defense in some non-specific way. The strategy behind all these interventions has been likened to kicking the television set to make it work: give the immune system a good jolt, the thinking goes, and its capacity to rid the body of cancer cells may increase. Exactly which component, or combination of components could account for the killing of tumor cells still remains essentially unknown. Even so, the tactic has had some real success, not only by the cancer immunologists but also by some alternative medicine practitioners.

Today, immunotherapies for cancer are focused on much more *specific* ways to battle tumor cells. The discovery of monoclonal antibodies has made this very attractive. With this spectacular technology, scientists now produce unlimited supplies of identical antibodies which can be made to target specific tumor antigens. This is a kind of 'cellular star-wars'. These monoclonal antibodies, in principle, home-in on cancer cells by recognizing their specific antigens. That triggers an immune attack to destroy the target cells, all the while ignoring normal cells which lack the particular cancer antigens. It is conceivable that the antibodies could even be made to carry-in their own toxic chemicals directly to the tumor. This sounds simple and *natural* enough but like so much of good *science*, it is freight with problems to solve and burdens to overcome.

Research in this area remains hot, and slow but steady progress is being made. At the same time, other scientists are actively pursuing the possibility of active immunotherapy with a vaccine, to provoke an immune response which can, in principle, provide cancer protection for selected patients at risk of disease. That would further authenticate the real value of modern science and medicine. More importantly, it could make a world of difference for many people in our world today.

AIDS. Immune deficiencies as a result of cancer or from extensive anticancer therapy are all examples of acquired immunodeficiency states. Other immunodeficiency disorders can also be inherited. Some children are born with defects in their immune systems. They lack one or more of its essential components. But without doubt, by far the most devastating and the most widespread immunodeficiency disorder today is the acquired immunodeficiency syndrome (AIDS). Since it was first recognized in 1981, it has become pandemic. The World Health Organization case estimates are now approaching 100 million people. AIDS now constitutes a serious threat to a significant portion of the world population. Over half of these are in central and southern Africa, but right here in North America many thousands of individuals have already died from the disease. Despite the massive investment of research dollars, both public and private, over 90% of all the diagnosed cases are expected to die from AIDS.

Again one must turn to good science for answers to the fundamental questions. It is hoped that a better understanding of the disease, better application of effective social, behavioral and public health measures to reduce transmission, a clearer and more definitive diagnosis of the disease, and, hopefully, some better therapeutic interventions and even potential vaccination against infection – all this and more will make the general outlook less depressing. This is a modern phenomenon demanding the best of *science* and no amount of simplistic *natural*, alternative therapies will blunt the threat. The scientific program over the past twenty years in understanding the cause and epidemiology of the disease was so rapid that it has no parallel with other infectious diseases. Even with this advanced present-day understanding, neither a vaccine nor a cure for AIDS are yet "around the corner".

We have gained a thorough understanding of HIV characteristics but we are still losing the war. HIV is a retrovirus. Like other viruses, it requires the synthetic apparatus of a host's cell for its replication. But as a retrovirus, it utilizes a unique system by which the ordinary flow of genetic information from DNA to RNA is reversed. A number of different mechanisms by which HIV functionally impairs and destroys CD4 (T4) cells has been proposed and exhaustively studied. Despite the enormous amount of information gathered in the past twenty years, the many residual gaps in our understanding of HIV infection and AIDS are reflected by the present lack of effective chemotherapy or immunotherapy and by the lack of an effective vaccine. A critical and elusive challenge remains the competence of the virus to survive by constant mutation.

The bottom line is that **there is presently no cure for AIDS,** although the exceptional antiviral agent zidovuzine (AZT) appears to hold the virus in check, at least for a time. Many other antiretroviral drugs are being tested, as are agents to bolster the immune system and agents to prevent or treat opportunistic infections. Research on vaccines to prevent the spread of AIDS is also under way. Again, **we can only rely on good *science* to unravel the mysteries of this global plague** and with its answers point a way forward in hope.

AUTOIMMUNITY.   AIDS represents in one sense, one extreme of what can go wrong with the immune system. For all intents and purpose, the defensive forces are overwhelmed and lose the war. It is dysfunction due to deficiency.

Autoimmune disorders represent, in a similar sense, the other extreme where the immune system becomes too aggressive and overzealous, and now it over-reacts to substances that it would normally ignore. It is a kind of hypersensitivity, similar to allergies. In the case of allergies, the immune system reacts to an external substance that would otherwise be harmless. With autoimmune disorders, the internal recognition apparatus breaks down and the immune system reacts to normal "self" body tissues. The normal control process, dictated by the T-suppressor cells, is disrupted and the dysfunction spreads. Now the body begins to manufacture antibodies (auto antibodies) and T-cells directed against the body's own constituents. Such antibodies are known as autoantibodies and they trigger cytotoxic immune damage or they form complexes with self antigen to activate the complement cascade and lead to tissue damage. The consequences of autoimmunity may vary from minimal to catastrophic, depending on the extend to which the integrity of self-tolerance has been affected. Not all autoantibodies are harmful, however, and some types appear to be integral to the immune system's regulatory scheme.

The causes of autoimmune disease are not exactly clear, but several factors are likely to be involved. These may include viruses and environmental factors such as exposure to sunlight, certain chemicals, and some drugs, all of which may damage or alter body cells so that they are no longer recognizable as self. Sex hormones may be important, too, since most autoimmune diseases are far more common in women than in men. Because autoimmune disorders and allergy are both considered hypersensitivity reactions, it is likely that a history of allergy indicates increase risk for autoimmunity too. Statistically, it has been linked to left handedness for no apparent reason. Heredity also appears to play a role. Autoimmune reactions, like many other immune responses, are influenced by the genes of the MHC since a high proportion of human patients with autoimmune disease have particular histocompatibility types.

Many types of therapies are being used to combat autoimmune disease. These include corticosteroids, immunosuppressive drugs developed as anticancer agents, radiation of the lymph nodes, and plasmapheresis, a sort of "blood washing" that removes diseased cells and harmful molecules from the circulation. In any case, it is a balancing act. The goal is to reduce the immune response against normal body tissue while leaving intact the immune response against micro-organism and abnormal tissues. The outcome varies with the specific disorder but in most cases, the disorders are chronic but controlled with good management.

There is an unusual irony illustrated here. Alternative practitioners and advocates of *natural* healing make a habit of pointing out that orthodox medicine focuses on symptomatic treatment, whereas they address the *root cause* of health problems. That may be a wise observation in the context of psycho-social and emotional issues, but in the area of organic illness such as a dysfunctional immune system (and autoimmunity, in particular) nothing could be further from the truth. Autoimmune disorders are quite often chronic conditions. Physicians struggle to manage patients with arthritis, lupus, juvenile-onset diabetes and the like, knowing that the root cause is elusive despite all the textbooks and research on autoimmunity. *They know so much that they appreciate how little they really know.* The immune systems is exceedingly complex. But then, because they find no cure for *the root cause*, the effectiveness of orthodox and allopathic management is more and more being questioned – not only by alternative practitioners, but now by the public at large.

In contrast, the public (thanks to the media culture, advertising and hectic lifestyles) seems to be demanding more and more, a version of instant health. In the absence of real solutions, quite often they are given a therapeutic version of 'fast food'. It appears to satisfy the appetite but does not fulfil the body's real need. There is no real cure for rheumatoid arthritis for example, and the best of all *natural* remedies provide nothing more than symptomatic relief. But those who make the exaggerated claims for their *natural* interventions and attribute their apparent solutions to a resolution of the real root cause, must obviously *know so little, that they know not how little they really do know.*

Clearly, we can learn from *nature*, but nature reveals her secrets to diligent, inquiring minds that pursue *science* and pay the price of real discovery.

We will explore one such breakthrough in the next chapter, one that could revolutionize our clinical management of the immune system at a fundamental level.

Chapter Five

BREAKTHROUGH
IN CELL-DEFENSE
A Major Discovery for the 21st Century

T his is a story of good science. It is a story of serendipity. As so often happens in science, diligent research in pursuit of some problem often leads investigators to unexpected findings, sometimes quite unrelated to the original question being examined. That's essentially what happened here.

It is the story of the celebrated scientist **Dr. Gustavo Bounous**, and how he stumbled on to a major breakthrough for the immune system. In a previous book by the same title as this chapter, we chronicled the life story of this eminent researcher and how he opened a door to the future of nutritional pharmacology.

Dr. Bounous was born in Luserna, Italy and graduated from Medical School at the University of Turin. He trained as a surgeon in Parma and then Genoa but after completing his residency, he moved to the United States in 1956 and began surgical research at the Indiana University Medical Center with Prof. Shumacher. His first contributions were in the patho-physiology of renal blood flow and hypertension. When his visa expired he was obliged to leave the U.S. and took up residency in Canada where he worked with the famed surgeon Prof. Fraser Gurd at the McGill University Surgical Research Unit. There he published numerous research papers on diverse subjects in the area of cardiovascular medicine and surgery.

Dr. Bounous' first major contribution to science and medicine really came about when he solved the patho-physiology of hemorrhagic shock. This was a serious challenge for a number of very ill patients (quite often seen post-operatively) who would hemorrhage, and despite receiving all the known appropriate fluid therapy and care, they would 'crash' and die almost precipitously. In 1964, Dr. Bounous stumbled upon the solution and was able to identify the relationship of intestinal metabolic changes to hemorrhagic enteritis and the barrier function of intestinal mucosa. In a nutshell, he found that when the lining of the intestine was deprived of oxygen, its essential protection from the digestive action of pancreatic secretions was lost and the enzymes would 'puncture a hole' in the bowel leading to peritonitis, septic shock and imminent death. For this seminal work, the young researcher was awarded the prestigious Medal of the Royal College of Physicians and Surgeons of Canada. As a further consequence, he was made a Career Investigator for the Medical Research Council of Canada, a privilege he retained for twenty five years until his recent retirement, despite the rigorous scrutiny of research review committees on a regular basis.

That discovery soon led Dr. Bounous to propose the use of 'predigested' foods which support the mucosa and at the same time, reduce the digestive enzymes in the gut. This he first called an 'Elemental Diet' in 1967, an idea which pushed him into the mainstream of the nutritional field but at right angles to the medical establishment. It would take about twenty years for this pioneering use of *diet or nutrition* to become standard practice in both prophylaxis and management of such serious medical conditions as hemorrhagic shock, radiation sickness, cancer chemotherapy or inflammatory bowel disease.

Dr. Bounous' unselfish and rather modest style, and his surgical research interest, both coupled with his knowledge and growing reputation of how nutrition affects the body *at the cellular level*, eventually attracted the right components that would lead him to make what is promising to become one of the most significant medical discoveries of the twentieth century.

On an otherwise uneventful day, Dr. Bounous received a package in the mail containing a fine, white powder – some milk whey concentrate, according to the accompanying letter. A European food company was facing a giant problem, causing much embarrassment and a corporate headache. As a milk by-product from cheese manufacture, this useless powder had been routinely dumped into the local rivers and streams. Unfortunately it seemed, the product was rich in nitrogen and local flora had overgrown and was threatening to clog the waterways.

That was a new major ecological challenge. Environmentalists and local governments were up in arms. Something had to be done. Because of his reputation, company officials turned to the medical/nutritional 'expert' to see if at the very least, there might be some better way to dispose of it.

Dr. Bounous fed the mysterious powder to a small group of mice to compare their response with a similar group fed a more normal maintenance diet. There was no qualitative difference in general appearance, growth, attitude or activity of the mice when fed with this non-specific whey powder. However, when challenged with T-cell dependent antigen, these mice produced more antibodies compared to the normal mice fed with the standard maintenance diets. This was reported in the *Journal of Infectious Diseases* in 1981.

DISCOVERIES

Dr. Bounous was soon introduced to an immunologist at McGill, Dr. Patricia Kongshavn. She had the laboratory, the animals and much expertise to accelerate this new field of interest. Their combined interest focused initially on the effect of dietary amino acids (protein building blocks) on immune reactivity. Later they would look at a variety of common dietary proteins. To measure the immune response, Kongshavn suggested they use two fairly standard methods.

i)   The Plaque Forming Cell (PFC) assay for *humoral immune responses* (antibody production). This method was used for assaying the immune response, as modified by Cunningham and Szenberg. Mice were injected intravenously (i.v.) with sheep red-blood-cells (sRBC) and then the spleen was assayed for plaque-forming-cells (PFC) five days after inoculation when the response was shown to peak.

ii)   Mitogen responses. The method described by Lapp and coworkers was used to test the mitogen response to different concentrations of phytohemagglutinin (PHA), concanavalin A (con A) and lipopolysaccharide (LPS) mitogens in the spleen, with or without stimulation with BCG mycobacterium. The PHA and Con A responses were indicative of the other fundamental component of the immune system i.e. the *cellular immune response*, while the LPS response measured the B cell responses.

The first results of Bounous and Kongshavn were more definitive for the negative effect of severe dietary restriction, particularly of some essential amino acids. They tentatively proposed that this caused a suppression of the production or function of some inhibitory cell such as a T-suppressor cell, while not affecting the influencing cell to the same degree.

But the question still remained. Was there some special dietary manipulation that could *positively* and *consistently* enhance the immune response? That was the question to prompt the design and execution of novel experiments in the field. Bounous and Kongshavn were in pursuit of an answer.

Immuno-enhancement

The pair turned to investigating various edible dietary proteins – including casein, lactalbumin or whey protein of milk, soy and wheat. Of these, lactalbumin uniquely enabled the mice to develop an immune response which was consistently greater than that for comparable mice which were fed the other protein diets.

Mice are the laboratory animals of choice in immunological research. They have afforded major advances in the understanding of the immune system, which has led to many applications in clinical medicine. They are mammals and therefore extrapolation can be made for application to humans. There is also a vast body of reference data for consistent comparison. They are available to scientists in select genetically identical strains, with defined phenotypic characteristics.

In a typical Bounous experiment, the mice would be purchased from the breeders at five or six weeks of age. They were housed in wire-bottomed cages to maintain a clean hygienic environment. They were fed by placing feedings (typically three times a week) in stainless-steel dispensers for continuous availability of the powder without spillage or contamination. Drinking water was usually available at all times. Various diets would be commenced at six to eight weeks of age and immunological studies initiated one, two or three weeks later. The mice were commonly fed in different but comparable dietary groups of ten or twelve each.

The effect of graded amounts of dietary lactalbumin (whey protein concentrate) (L) and casein (C) hydrolyzates on the immune responsiveness of two different strains of mice, was investigated by measuring both the specific humoral immune response to sheep red blood cells (sRBC) and the nonspecific splenic cell responsiveness to mitogens after BCG stimulation. The nutritional efficiency of these diets was similar at both 12 and 28% amino acid levels. The immune responses of mice fed the L diets were found to be significantly greater than those of mice fed the corresponding C diets, especially at the 28% level. Furthermore in mice fed the L diet, increasing the concentration of amino acid in the diet from 12 to 28% greatly enhanced immune responsiveness by both parameters measured. In the C-fed mice, a comparable enhancement of mitogen responsiveness with increasing amino acid level of diet was seen, but there was no change in the humoral immune response. These dietary effects on immune responsiveness were remarkably similar in both mice strains tested.

"Lactalbumin" was the term traditionally used to describe the *group* of milk proteins that remain soluble in "milk serum" or whey after precipitation of casein at pH 4.6 and 20°C, as in the normal manufacture of cheese. The major components of the whey protein mixture were actually determined to be beta-lactoglobulin, alpha-lactalbumin, serum albumin and immunoglobulin.

Bounous and Kongshavn demonstrated unequivocally that mice fed diets containing any one of the major *components* of "lactalbumin," currently called "whey protein concentrate", or "isolate", in the concentration of 20% by weight in the diet, developed immune responses to sheep red blood cells which were inferior to that of mice fed a diet containing 20% by weight of the mixture (lactalbumin). Hence, the assumption was made that the immunoenhancing effect of lactalbumin was dependent on the overall amino acid pattern resulting from the contribution of all its protein components.

There was no equivalent substitute: not free amino acids, neither casein, soy, wheat or corn protein, egg albumin, beef or fish protein, *Spirulina maxima* or *Scenedesmus* algae protein, or Purina mouse chow. These were all tried and they all failed. Only with the whey powder could the immunoenhancing effect be manifest after two weeks and persist for at least eight weeks of dietary treatment. Mixing lactalbumin with casein or soy protein in a 20% diet formula significantly enhanced the immune response in comparison to that of mice which were fed diets containing either 20% soy protein or casein. Obviously, whey protein somehow enhanced immune response.

Increased Resistance

Very early in their efforts, Bounous and Kongshaven decided to inoculate laboratory animals orally with bacteria (*Salmonella typhimurium* and later with *Streptococcus pneumoniae, type 3* and *Escherichia coli),* to see if there was any increased protection from feeding them lactalbumin. The mice chosen, though virtually identical before innoculation, had widely varying fates: some died, others became sick, but those fed milk whey concentrate appeared brighter and more healthy as they scampered about in their cage. Obviously the whey powder worked ... but the two research scientists still did not know why. Why would a whey protein concentrate have any such immuno-enhancing effect? What special property might this powder have? They were intrigued and challenged.

In a follow up study, Bounous and Kongshavn collaborated with Dr. Osmond, another colleague at McGill, to examine the genesis of B lymphocytes in the bone marrow, using two different strains of mice. The findings indicated that the observed effects of altered dietary protein type on humoral immune responsiveness were not exerted centrally on the rate of primary B-lymphocyte production in the bone marrow, but more likely, reflected changes either in the functional responsiveness of the B-lymphocytes themselves or in the processes leading to their activation and differentiation in the peripheral lymphoid tissues.

Because minerals and trace metals including zinc and copper had been found to influence the immune response, it was necessary to eliminate the possibility that the dietary proteins were influencing their rate of absorption or bioavailability. That evidence was clear. A previous study had also shown that the principal factor responsible for the observed differential effect of dietary lactalbumin and casein on humoral immunity was not the availability or concentration of single amino acids but rather the composite effect of the specific amino acid distribution in the protein.

Later, the *immodulatory effects of dietary whey proteins in mice* were also confirmed independently by Wang and Watson at the CSIRO Division of Animal Health in Australia. Again they showed that ingestion of bovine milk whey proteins, either as a supplement in an adequately balanced commercial diet or as the only protein source in a balanced diet, consistently enhanced secondary humoral antibody responses when compared with other protein sources such as soybean protein isolate and ovine colostral whey proteins. The effects were again unrelated solely to the nutritional factors.

Such independent confirmation is always to be expected in the reporting of good *science*. In fact, it is a hallmark: in different hands, at different times, in different places, with different samples – all giving the same results! That is called reproducibility, anything less is NOT science.

An adequate intake of essential amino acids is necessary because surplus amino acids are not stored and, for protein synthesis to proceed, all the indispensable amino acids must be present simultaneously in the extracellular pool. With regard to the humoral immune response, clonal expansion and antibody production require rapid protein synthesis, so that amino acid restriction will inevitably interfere with these functions. *But why is the 'distribution' and not the 'adequacy' the point at issue with these mice diets*? Questions like this not only haunted Drs. Bounous and Kongshavn but it stimulated their creative minds. One experiment led to the other. Every result prompted a different question and every question generated a new idea for experimental design. That's also the normal process of *science*.

Anti-tumor

The real opportunity to study any possible cancer effects of lactalbumin came through the proximity of a cancer research laboratory on the same ninth floor of the McGill University Surgical Clinic. Just down the corridor, two young researchers, Drs. Papenburg and Fleiszer, had utilized a method to evaluate the effects of 1, 2 - dimethylhydrazine on the development of intestinal tumors. They were very willing to cooperate. Dr. Bounous and his new colleagues therefore set out to determine the effect of whey protein in diets on the development of a chemically-induced type of murine tumor.

In the earlier studies, the immunoenhancing property was found to be maximized at a 20% concentration of whey protein in the diet. That meant 20gm whey protein per 100gm diet. In fact, they found that raising the protein level of either whey protein itself, or casein, soy or wheat protein in the diet above 20% failed to enhance the immune response of the host beyond the values observed with the 20gm protein per 100gm diet. In addition, at this level, most proteins including those used in the test formula diets, supplies the minimum requirement of all indispensable amino acids for the growing mouse. So they chose a 20% protein concentration for the cancer study.

1,2 – Dimethylhydrazine had been demonstrated by Rogers and Nauss and by Alinen to be a convenient potent carcinogen which produced rodent carcinomas of the colon in a reproducible manner. In other words, it could be used as an animal model of colon cancer relevant to human disease. Others had previously shown that fiber, fat and the level of dietary protein could be either protective (fiber) or promotive (fat, protein) in dimethylhydrazine – induced colon carcinogenesis. The tumors were characteristically located in the distal bowel and long term exposure to the carcinogen was required before the lesions appeared. (Parenthetically, colon cancer in mice is also a convenient model because the response to chemotherapy is similar to human cancers.)

Dr. Bounous therefore chose dimethylhydrazine and thirty mice of a specific strain, for the classic study of the effect of his new amazing, immunoenhancing whey protein concentrate. He chose to divide the mice into three equal groups of ten which were individually numbered and housed in similar cages with five animals per cage. The mice were obtained at six to-eight weeks of age and then started on the test diets three weeks prior to commencing carcinogen treatment.

Three test diets were prepared with 20% of either whey protein concentrate or casein, or the usual Purina mouse chow (estimated 23% protein). The only variable in the two purified diets was the type of protein. They also included 56% of a protein-free diet powder containing corn syrup, corn oil, tapioca starch, vitamins and minerals, 18% cornstarch, 2% wheat fiber, 0.5% vit-iron premix, 2.65% potassium chloride and 0.84% sodium chloride (salt).

The carcinogen was prepared by dissolving the powdered chemical in normal saline to a concentration of 15mg/100ml with the pH adjusted to 6.9-7.0 using saturated sodium hydroxide. Carcinogen solutions were used on the same day as they were prepared. The mice were fed the different diets for three weeks initiation and the test diets were maintained throughout the duration of the experiment. They were injected subcutaneously with a weekly dose of 15mg dimethylhydrazine per kilogram of body weight for twenty four weeks.

The animals were sacrificed four weeks after their 24th injection. Their colons were removed, opened longitudinally, fecal contents removed, and the colons then weighed and their length measured. Tumor burden was assessed both by the number of tumors and the sum of the vertical and horizontal tumor diameters of all grossly visible tumors.

To Dr. Bounous' surprise, he found that whey-protein-fed animals developed significantly fewer tumors per animal and moreover, the tumor area development was also significantly less. This was seen despite the similarity in body weight curves, apparently ruling out conventional nutritional factors to account for the observed differences in the development of tumors.

It was well known at that time that the incidence and size of tumors were influenced by the immune system. In the advanced state of disease in which Bounous also made plaque-forming-cell (PFC) measurements, the humoral immune response was greatly reduced in all three dietary groups in the classic cancer study. The measurements, nevertheless, reflected the pattern of humoral immune response in relation to food protein type that they had earlier seen in their laboratory on healthy mice. It was therefore conceivable that, particularly in the early phase of tumor development, the protein-related differences in immune reactivity among the three dietary groups could have influenced the observed difference in tumor development that Dr. Bounous had just seen with his very eyes.

Dr. Bounous went on to publish these amazing observations in a classic paper published in the *Journal of Clinical and Investigative Medicine* (1988). He coauthored it with several of his colleagues: They were bold enough to give the paper its provocative title claim: **"Dietary whey protein inhibits the development of dimethyl-hydrazine-induced malignancy."**

It was now made public for the establishment to see. **This is the critical path of** *science*. **One must submit one's work to peer review and publish results for critical analysis by every interested expert in the field. There is no room for veiled secrets or hidden agendas. The real truth about** *nature* **is singular and every valid conclusion will withstand the test of time and talent.** These amazing results would be later confirmed in *rats* by a different group of Australian investigators. Again, such confirmation is the hallmark of good research.

Anti - aging

Equally significant, the doctors became convinced that the whey protein concentrate may possess both prophylactic and therapeutic value. In these early classic studies, Bounous and his team had also noted coincidentally that the whey-fed mice not only had an enhanced immune response and an apparent anti-tumor activity, but in general they fared better and showed better survival rates. What did this mean in effect? Was it as basic an observation as an anti-aging phenomenon? Those were provocative questions.

Studies performed at the Eppley Cancer Center in Nebraska were consistent with Bounous's earlier findings on the immunoenhancing effect of dietary lactalbumin. Survival (resistance to spontaneous diseases) of *hamsters* of both sexes, measured over a twenty week period of feeding from four weeks of age, was best with a 20% lactalbumin diet, in comparison with a 20% methionine and cysteine supplemented casein diet. Body weight gains were similar in both groups to suggest overall nutritional protein equivalency. In addition too, in lifetime feeding studies, the mean and maximal longevity of female and male hamsters fed 10, 20 and 40% lactalbumin diets was increased in comparison with those fed commercial laboratory feed with estimated 24% protein from various sources. Survival was again best with the 20% lactalbumin diet. In the males, longevity increased by 50%. No relationship was noted between food intake, maximal weight, and longevity.

Again, the lactalbumin diet increased survival and longevity beyond that of 'control' animals fed either of two nutritionally adequate reference diets, thus enhancing life expectancy beyond the limits traditionally assumed to be "normal". Bounous found that in one group of mice, whey protein concentrate actually increased their life spans by thirty percent over three months.

Could this then all add up to a general anti-aging effect of Bounous's whey protein concentrate? Was it truly protective and life-sustaining at least for these experimental animals?

Medical Dynamite

At first, Bounous and coworkers found a surprising immuno-enhancing effect in the mice, then increased bacterial resistance, then an anti-tumor effect and now a possible anti-aging observation. Could they be handling 'medical dynamite' indeed? The answers were not yet clear.

These dietary investigations were still very much on the outskirts of usual scientific interest, but they continued to occupy Bounous and his colleagues as they pursued the *science* of it all. In 1981 their report, *"The Effect of Dietary Amino Acid on the Growth of Tumors"* had hardly caused a ripple in medicine's collective consciousness. The nutritional substrate was too ordinary. It held no pharmacological appeal. **Even today, medicine still has not widely accepted the fact that nutrition undeniably plays an enormous role in both prevention and treatment of major diseases.**

After almost a decade of research, this whey protein concentrate had indeed proven to be more than just a nuisance by-product of the cheese manufacturing industry. It was now showing promise for unexpected clinical use, at least for medical research. In the best case scenario, it could have far-reaching implications in clinical practice. What was originally a search for a practical solution to an environmental hazard, was now threatening to become, to some degree at least, an elixir for the human condition. But this would remain nothing more than a prospect, until a more fundamental understanding of the observed effects of the whey protein could be elucidated. That was the puzzle crying out desperately for solution.

EUREKA

In a chance meeting over coffee one morning in their research department, a frustrated Dr. Bounous had a fateful discussion with a young brilliant researcher, Dr. Gerald Batist. Although providence had placed their laboratories only yards apart, the meeting of the minds was reserved for this moment in time. They greeted each other that day for the first time. As you would expect of avid researchers, they quickly gravitated to shop talk. It turned out that this particular colleague was working on something called **glutathione** and some possible role in cancer.

Dr. Batist, who was already established in his field, proceeded to explain how cysteine, a protein building block found in whey, *could* implicate his pet molecule glutathione, the all-important tripeptide synthesized inside the cell for its own protection, and this could lead to immuno-enhancement and more.

Could it be as simple as that? One important molecule? A glutathione connection?

What Batist had just proposed in this chance meeting was as simple as it was profound. Whey must have some unique, or at least special characteristics that could influence cellular *glutathione*. A lot of research had already been done on that amazing cellular constituent. It was a biochemical gem made inside the cell with a critical role in cell-defense. But no progress had ever been made in its desirably safe, effective or convenient control or manipulation until this time. Perhaps what Batist had suggested could become a key to unlock a treasure of physiological and clinical possibilities. These would hold far-reaching implications of which immunenhancement with increased resistance to infectious pathogens, increased resistance to chemically induced tumors and possible anti-aging effects were only just a beginning.

"Dr. Batist was *the* expert on *the* subject that Dr. Bounous needed to know about. He was the only one at McGill then working on glutathione. There he was, working forty or fifty yards away at the other end of the corridor, working on the other half of Dr. Bounous' experiments. He had the missing link all that time and neither of them knew. They had been so close and yet so far.

They had an immediate handle on the problem. At least they could verify his suggestion one way or the other. Dr. Bounous proceeded to look again at his whey protein chemistry, and saw that whey indeed contained the cysteine amino acid precursor of glutathione. Some unique property of the whey must make it particularly effective. The enormity of the implications – *why, **this whey protein did lead straight to a single main element so vital to cell defense!***

PROOF

But new knowledge to a critical researcher's mind always stimulates new thoughts and consequently new questions. This leads to the design of new experiments to gain more knowledge which of course, starts the cycle all over again. Again, that's the basic scientific paradigm.

The immediate challenge was naturally to seek to prove Dr. Batist's theory that the immuno-enhancing property of dietary whey protein, in mice at least, was mediated through the ubiquitous glutathione. The definitive study set out to measure the immune response by plaque-forming cell assay and simultaneously, the splenic glutathione levels. They used three dietary regimes: whey protein, casein and a supplemented casein with added free L-cysteine, in adequate amounts to mimic the cysteine content of the whey protein. They also tried to confirm any possible impact of whey protein on splenic glutathione by measuring the immune response in the presence of buthionine sulfoximine (BSO) which blocks the glutathione synthesis. Furthermore, they investigated the effect of each major component of the whey protein concentrate on the plaque forming cells' response. They measured quantitatively the concentration of glutathione with an ultraviolet spectrophotometer. This was essentially the method described by Anderson and afforded real tissue values for glutathione in micromoles per gram of wet tissue.

The results were clear. The similar weight gain for each diet group indicated similar food consumption and similar serum protein values were obtained. However, after challenging mice with an immune stimulus and measuring the specific humoral immune response to sheep red blood cells, the response was almost 500% as much for the mice which were fed the whey protein diet compared to the casein diet and the cysteine - enriched casein diet.

The results could not be related to some fortuitous milk protein allergy or some other manifestation of oral immunization. Again, the type of protein in the diet was found to have little or no effective difference on all the other parameters they examined, including body growth, food consumption, serum protein, minerals and trace metals, and circulating white cells (lymphocytes). The difference was therefore not one of "adequacy" of essential amino acids. It had to be in protein type, structure or function.

The only significant effect of protein type was a change in the amino acid profile in the plasma, which conformed to the amino acid composition of the ingested protein, *except for cysteine.* Again, despite the eight-fold higher difference in cysteine content in the whey protein diet, the plasma level of cysteine was not different in the whey protein diet - fed mice from that of the casein diet-fed counterparts. And not surprising, dietary cysteine is known to be the rate limiting precursor for the synthesis of glutathione. Therefore cysteine became highly suspect as the critical variable in the diets.

In the classic experiment by Bounous and Batist, the results demonstrated a significant difference between the effects of casein and whey protein diets on the splenic glutathione concentration during the oxygen-requiring, antigen – driven clonal expansion of the lymphocytes, and following that expansion, in the development of humoral immunity. This could reflect the ability of the lymphocytes of the whey protein-fed mice to offset any potential oxidative damage, thus allowing them to respond more fully to the antigenic stimulus. The efficiency of dietary cysteine in inducing supernormal and immune - effective glutathione levels was apparently superior when delivered in the whey protein rather than as free cysteine. Blockage of the glutathione synthesis (with BSO inhibiting a special synthetase enzyme) produced a four to five fold drop in the immune response in whey protein-fed mice, just as the Batist theory had suggested. And the immunoenhancing effect is maintained when the whey protein is used and not when free cysteine is added to the casein. Obviously, the specific amino acid profile of whey protein or a cysteine containing peptide is an important factor in determining the fate of ingested cysteine.

So, the theory which was readily advanced by Dr. Batist over coffee that morning when Dr. Bounous happened to sit beside him, was now supported by experimental observations. As Dr. Batist was also quick to point out, glutathione was known to be central in a wide variety of reactions - among them, for example, detoxifying potentially toxic and/or carcinogenic xenobiotics. Thus, they had only just touched the surface. The impact of whey protein by increasing the splenic glutathione levels should have potential implications far beyond the humoral immune response system alone.

This was a watershed realization. Dr. Bounous had found the door to open new vistas of clinical possibilities. It was glutathione, the intracellular tripeptide that played such a central role. But more importantly, he realized that he had found the key to open that door. It was as simple and as common as the special dietary whey protein he was studying. He was just beginning to appreciate the potential "medical dynamite" sitting in his research lap.

"Eureka!"

SERENDIPITY

With this understanding of the central role of glutathione in cell-defense and his clear observations that his 20% whey protein diet could effectively raise (or perhaps optimize) the intracellular glutathione levels, Dr. Bounous redoubled his research efforts. There were so many more questions arising almost daily. There was the temptation to jump at short-cut applications before a more thorough understanding of the fundamental mechanisms. But a keen scientist all his life, Bounous refused to be side-tracked from his deepest longing, his real motivation. He must find answers to questions of physiology and biochemistry. If he could only find more answers to the fundamentals. So, that meant back to the laboratory. Back to designing new experiments and diligently making more observations. He was sure that *nature* would inevitably yield some other secret that remained obscure, if not to him, then certainly to someone just as daring.

Then suddenly, inexplicably ... the unthinkable happened. The whey concentrate simply ceased to be biologically effective. It seemed to have lost all its previous bioactivity. Try as he might, Dr. Bounous no longer found it possible to make any of his experiments succeed. He could not reproduce the previous results. Nothing worked as before. That is a scientist's nightmare: The inability to reproduce results. The nutritional efficiency of the whey proteins had not changed. But there was no longer immuno-enhancement. No bacterial resistance. No tumor inhibition. No anti-aging effect. No more significant effects. Period. Ironically, now that the scientist at last had discovered why the whey protein worked, suddenly it failed. Trial after laboratory trial failed. Suddenly, it seemed, research had reached an impasse. Experimental results all turned negative. As we emphasized earlier, the true hallmark of good *science*, is always reproducibility. Any experiment that's trustworthy must be consistently verifiable, in different hands at different times, given the same conditions. Bounous knew that maxim and he himself would insist on it. Therefore the onus was on him. He could not retreat now.

One night, while tuning out after a day's hard work and alone as usual, Dr. Bounous idly watched a Swiss television program in which two men discussed gourmet cooking. One chef commented that cheese no longer tasted as good as it once did, and the other man replied that when the government required pasteurization temperatures to be raised, it lessened the quality of cheeses. There was more. During the conversation between the two participants, Bounous learned that European milk and cheese producers had been required to raise pasteurization temperatures from seventy two degrees centigrade to seventy-eight degrees, to provide added safety to all European milk and cheese products. This was apparently in response to a previous outbreak of salmonella in France. Bounous and his partner Kongshavn, in the early days you remember, had studied the effect of feeding whey to the mice and noting if their resistance to salmonellosis was altered.

The mention of Salmonella got Dr. Bounous' attention, but that was not the real issue.

Long ago, when he first dug in to study the chemistry of proteins, Dr. Bounous had learned one fact that apparently was now proving to be a major key to the puzzle: the delicate cystine residue in whey protein becomes denatured after it receives a certain amount of heat. *Those few degrees of temperature had made his whey proteins incapable of enhancing glutathione in the cells of mice and possibly men.* The higher temperature had probably disturbed the cystine structure, somehow or other. The cystine structure? What's that?

Every high school student today will probably know the story of *The Double Helix*. This is the simple model of Nobel prize winners Watson and Crick who first in 1956 beat out Linus Pauling with the proposal for a three-dimensional description of the DNA molecule. That model consists of two complementary helices, each of which represents the structure of a polymeric strand of nucleic acids, and which are held together by a limited number of specific base – pairs which form intra molecular bridges. That all-important three dimensional structure, as simple as it is - and verified by x-ray crystallography and much, much more - forms the basis for the genetic code and explains in meaningful comprehensible terms, a mechanism for such important biological processes as protein synthesis, cell replication, information transfer, cloning and so much more. It is the foundation of modern genetics and cell biology.

That is the sublime example of a general property of biologically active macromolecules. They all have specific composition and structure. That structure derives from the composition of linear repeating units, each of specific geometry, which then give rise to a natural conformation or shape of the final three-dimensional structure. Many important processes are determined by the critical tertiary structure of the complete macromolecule and often their associated units. That explains for example, the ability of hemoglobin to carry oxygen in reversible association in the blood-stream. It is the basis of all enzymatic processes which show a specific key-and-lock stereochemistry, whose unique efficiency leads all inquiring minds to awe and wonder.

That night watching television, Dr. Bounous came to the realization, however serendipitously, that in the production of whey protein concentrate, a change in temperature of just a few degrees during pasteurization of the milk and prior to the casein separation for cheese manufacturing, had had a profound impact on the product. This is not enough heat change to cause separation by boiling off some volatile ingredient or breaking up molecules into various fragments. But it is just adequate to cause labile inter- or intra-molecular bridges to fall apart. In addition, some crucial heat labile whey proteins could be denatured, hence lost in the curd. Just a few degrees change in pasteurization temperature was enough to denature the essential protein structures. From batch to batch, a change in preparation conditions – just a few degrees, no more – was all it took to reap havoc in the laboratory. The critical proteins fell apart as it were, and lost that essential bioactivity that had excited Bounous when he observed the amazing effects on his whey protein-fed mice.

We now understand that the essential bioactivity of Dr. Bounous' unique whey protein concentrate was dependent upon a critical concentration of three bioactive proteins contained in the milk serum and which are all sensitive to heat in a liquid base. They are:

✓ LACTOFERRIN
✓ SERUM ALBUMIN, and
✓ ALPHA LACTALBUMIN

These proteins contain exceptional amounts of **cysteine**, the critical rate-limiting **molecular** precursor of glutathione. More importantly, it is the **form** of the cysteine which is present that is so critical. The cysteine does occur in pairs in different parts of the protein chains. **Cystine** is the name of this so-called dipeptide unit. Note the different spelling of **cystine** (*the dipeptide*) and **cysteine** (*the amino acid*). In fact, cysteine occurs in two different dipeptide units, i.e. cystine (cys-cys) and glutamyl cysteine (glu-cys). These dipeptides are held together by the disulfide (S-S) bridges which can be kept undenatured under stringent conditions and even remain undigested for absorption into cells. Therein lies the Breakthrough.

When undenatured, these proteins contain almost the same number of cystine residues per total amino acid. Hence, as Table 4 shows, in serum albumin, there are 17 cystine residues per 66,000 MW molecule, and six glutamylcystine (Glu-Cys) dipeptides: In lactoferrin, there are 17 cystine residues per 77,000 MW molecule, and four Glu-Cys dipeptides: And in alpha-lactalbumin, there are four cystine residues per 14,000 MW molecule. Conversely, casein, the predominant bovine (cow's milk) protein contains only 0-2 cysteine residues per molecule. Another milk protein beta-lactoglobulin has only two cystine residues per 18,400 MW molecule, and IgG1, the predominant immunoglobulin in cow's milk serum, only four disulphide bridges (cystine) per 166,000 MW molecule.

In addition, it has been demonstrated that the Glu-Cys precursors of GSH can easily enter the cell to be synthesized into GSH. Interestingly, the Glu-Cys dipeptide is an exclusive feature of the only obligatory foods in the early life of mammals and oviparous species, i.e., milk

Table 4.   PROTEIN COMPOSITION OF
             COW'S AND HUMAN MILK

| Protein | Composition (g/L) | | Cystine/ Molecule |
	Cow's Milk	Human Milk	
Casein	26	3.2	0*
Beta-lactoglobulin	3.2	Negligible	2
Alpha-lactalbumin	1.2	2.8	4
Serum albumin	0.4	0.6	17
Lactoferrin	0.14	2.0	17
Total cystine (mol/L)	8.19×10^{-4}	13.87×10^{-4}	
Total cystine	6.0	38.7	

* Casein has 0 to 2 cysteine/molecule

and egg white respectively. Throughout the digestive – absorptive process, the other co-existing protein fractions of whey (milk serum) influence the rate of release of the glutathione precursors into the blood. This also affords the bio-availability of these crucial ingredients. Uniquely so. Therein again lies the Breakthrough.

IMMUNOCAL™

Dr. Bounous and his colleagues remained focused on their research and had little interest in commercializing this breakthrough discovery. That was until they went in search of new laboratory space and facilities and met a successful business man and real estate developer who was fascinated by the nature of their work. They connected and soon with new financing available, research intensified and method-of-use patents were secured. The original whey protein concentrate (lactalbumin) was commercialized as the unique product called Immunocal™ by the new company, Immunotec Research Limited, of which Dr. Bounous himself became the Director of Research and Development. The entrepreneurs believed that what they were about could transcend the mere commercial interests to address genuine human needs. They were totally convinced of the astounding health-giving benefits of the biologically active Immunocal™ that Bounous had developed and they committed to complete their mission.

There was a lot more work to be done, especially in human clinical trials, but they were buoyed by their understanding of the fundamentals by this time. Fig. 3 illustrates the simplified process by which Immunocal™ releases cystine or glutamyl cysteine in the small intestine. After transport in the blood plasma, these cysteine dipeptides effectively cross the cell's membrane. Inside the cell, the dipeptide is cleaved to afford the amino acid cysteine precursor which can then be utilized for glutathione synthesis.

The availability of cysteine within the cell is the apparent rate-limiting factor in the synthesis of glutathione to replenish the cell's store during the immune response or after oxidative stress. Therefore the challenge is to make cysteine available inside the cell for increased synthesis of glutathione on demand.

FIGURE 3.

**Synthesis of glutathione: the cell's own antioxidant.
"Immunocal™ as a cysteine delivery system"**

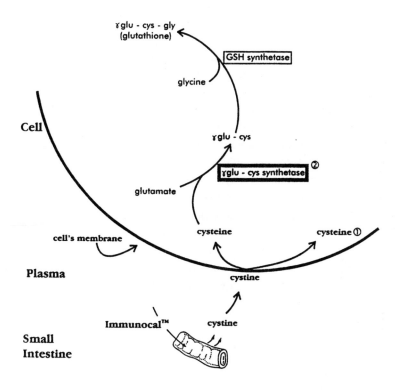

① Same pathway as the other identical molecule

② Inhibited by glutathione levels above normal

These facts had all come together. There was complete consistency at last. Glutathione was still the door. The unique whey protein concentrate was still the key. But it could only turn the door knob if the delicate structure of the **cysteine dipeptides** was intact. Now the fundamentals were clear:

- *Glutathione* is the key to the increased immune response, increased bacterial resistance, anti-tumor and anti-aging effects observed in mice.
- These cysteine dipeptides are the *effective* natural glutathione precursors.
- They remain *undigested* from specific dietary proteins.
- They (unlike glutathione itself) remain *stable* in the circulation and efficiently *cross* the cell membrane barrier to deliver their invaluable cysteine *inside*.
- They have immune system effects *independent* of their nutritional (protein source) contribution.
- They are the *essential* ingredients that produce significant, rapid glutathione replenishment in lymphocytes during the GSH-depleting immune response in the mice.
- They produce the moderate but sustained *increase* in organ/tissue glutathione of old mice following long term administration.
- They alone prove to be *safe, effective* and *convenient* for that purpose.
- Furthermore, only Immunocal™, *the whey protein concentrate of Dr. Bounous' discovery could deliver them.*
- They are **provided in nature** in as common a protein source as the whey derived from milk (nature's goldmine and as we shall see, in mother's breast milk too), and they are **preserved by science** only with careful, stringent technology.

Even after making all these new interesting observations and gaining an understanding of the mechanisms involved, Dr. Bounous and his colleagues did not quite grasp the significance of what they were about. It was only as their published papers began to circulate that other researchers, especially clinicians, began to show interest because of the relevance of their own fields of interest. That began to throw the door wide open and it became apparent that they were at the crest of a new wave in health and wellness, and even in therapeutics – one that was to become known as 'the Glutathione Revolution.' That's the subject of the next chapter.

Chapter Six

THE GLUTATHIONE REVOLUTION
Re-Thinking Medicine & Health

To appreciate the significance of Dr. Bounous' discovery of a safe, effective and convenient way to modulate cellular glutathione levels, one must grasp the importance of glutathione in the human body.

Glutathione was discovered by De-Rey-Pailliade in 1888 but it took one hundred years to come to center stage of the medical world. In the past two decades there has been a literal explosion of literature on the subject in the technical journals. In the past three years alone, a list of more than 5,000 such articles appeared and in just over a decade, that figure rises to more than 20,000. That information is now filtering down and out, and will soon make 'glutathione' a household word just like 'vitamins' or 'cholesterol' has become. At the same time, medical researchers in almost every clinical discipline are now obliged to address the fundamental question of how the levels of glutathione inside cells affect the pathophysiology of whatever disease process or health promotion they are focused on. Alternative practitioners are also eager to exploit this development because as central a cellular component as glutathione is proving to be, one can use a most *natural* intervention (select whey proteins) to modulate this critical parameter, without sophisticated diagnostics or specialized therapeutics and without any unnatural consequences. It represents a secret of nature as fundamental and as common as an obligatory provision in mother's breast milk.

What a unique meeting point for *science, nature* and *health*!

Indeed, glutathione could not be more central to health, and its importance in both prevention and disease management could hardly be exaggerated. In a word, it is the most critical defensive molecule *inside* human cells. Our cells depend on it and so does our life. Without it, those cells would soon be overwhelmed by oxidative stress, the liver and kidneys would literally clog up from the accumulation of toxins, our immune system would shut down and we would have no resistance to bacteria, viruses or cancer. As if that were not bad enough, the other systems like vitamins and enzymes, and even the DNA of the genetic code itself would fail to function properly, and no compensation would be possible. You get the picture.

Scientists are now beginning to appreciate the value of cell-defense per se and of glutathione in particular. In most medical schools today, the immune system is taught at the system level (how the body as a whole protects itself); or at the organ level (how the liver or spleen or bone marrow do their jobs in self-defense); or even at the cellular level (how specialized T-cells mount the cellular cytotoxic response and B-cells produce effective antibodies in the humoral response, and how the whole scheme is orchestrated by lymphokines and surface markers etc.). But hardly is the immune system focused on the most important level of all – at the *intra*cellular level. Healthy individual cells make up healthy organs which afford healthy bodies. Cells defend themselves against attack. They have enemies on the inside, molecules destined for their destruction. The critical defensive molecule *inside* the cell is this same glutathione. It is indeed the principal common protector against known common *intracellular* pathological mechanisms: oxidation, free radical formation, toxic chemical damage, and genetic mutation.

How much more central could glutathione be? But before we go on to describe the clinical significance (and the health importance too), we should quickly review some of the fundamentals regarding glutathione itself.

STRUCTURE AND FUNCTION

Glutathione (GSH) is a ubiquitous tripeptide molecule, consisting of three amino acids joined together. These are cysteine, glutamic acid and glycine — three of the twenty two amino acids which comprise the building blocks of all known proteins. In general, the *amino*-end of one amino acid combines with the *acid*-end of another to form a peptide bond with the elimination of water. Chains of amino acids are called proteins. The order of amino acids and the arrangement in space of each peptide bond define some specific structural features of all proteins and oligopeptides (a few amino acids in sequence) that relate to their function.

Glutathione is only synthesized *inside* cells, in a series of steps catalysed by specific enzymes. The *rate-limiting enzyme* is called γ-glutamyl cysteine synthetase since it joins the glutamic acid and cysteine residues, and the presence of intracellular cysteine is the *rate - limiting substrate*. Fig. 4 shows a simplified reaction scheme.

It is most significant that the key amino acid that comprises GSH has a so-called thiol (sulfhydryl) group i.e. – S-H. That is the basis for its abbreviated short form, GSH. The hydrogen atom attached to the sulfur is practically labile and it is this reversible transfer of hydrogen, which itself has an affinity for oxygenated (or oxidized) species, that gives it a powerful anti-oxidant capacity. It typically neutralizes any common oxygenated threat that comes across its path, so to speak. GSH is by far the most prevalent and active intracellular thiol, or intracellular antioxidant for that matter.

The role of oxygen in aerobic respiration is indispensable to cellular integrity and health but at the same time, normal cellular metabolism and exposure to the environment produces a number of reactive oxygen compounds inside each cell. Numerous mechanisms exist to prevent or treat the possible injurious events that can be triggered by these hyper-active oxygenated intermediates, which include oxy-, hydroxy- and peroxy-radicals, peroxides and superoxides. Recent focus on these degenerative processes have led scientists to stress the critical importance of so-called 'antioxidants' in the normal course of metabolism. For example, high interest has been generated in the actions of vitamins C and E, lipoic acid, melatonin, coenzyme Q10 and now increasingly, in glutathione. **Amongst the various antioxidant mechanisms, the "glutathione antioxidant system" is the leading cellular defense**. The GSH participates directly in the destruction of reactive oxygen compounds and it also maintains in the reduced (active) forms, other antioxidants such as ascorbate (vitamin C) and tocopherol (vitamin E). It is noteworthy that none of these important but lesser antioxi-

Figure 4.   The Glutathione Synthesis Challenge

GLUTATHIONE (GSH) :   A Tripeptide (3 amino acids)
γ - GLU - CYSH - GLY

gamma-glutamic acid   cysteine   glycine

GLUTATHIONE SYNTHESIS (inside the cell)

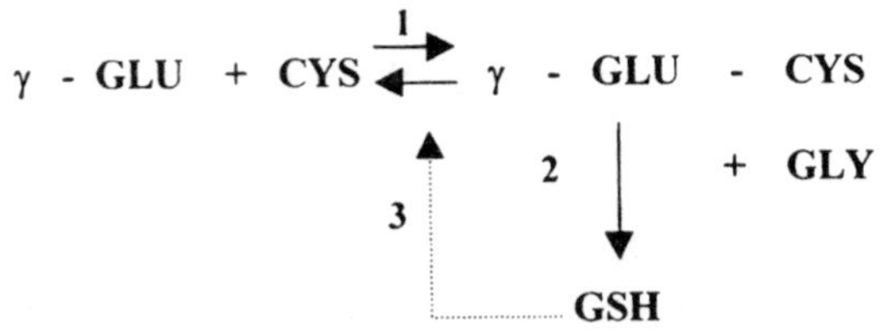

$$\gamma - GLU + CYS \underset{\longleftarrow}{\overset{1}{\longrightarrow}} \gamma - GLU - CYS$$

$$2 \downarrow + GLY$$

$$3 \uparrow$$

$$GSH$$

Reaction 1 is catalyzed by the enzyme γ - glutamylcysteine
   synthetase.
Reaction 2 is catalyzed by the enzyme GSH synthetase.
Reaction 3 is feedback inhibition by GSH, limiting its over-
   production

   The availability of cysteine within the cell is the apparent rate
limiting factor in the synthesis of glutathione to replenish the cell's stor
during the immune response or after oxidative stress. Therefore, th
challenge is to make cysteine available inside the cell for increase
synthesis of glutathione on demand.

dants occur naturally in the cell. **Glutathione is the only** *endogeneous*
antioxidant, complementary to superoxide dismutase (SOD). All others are obtained from the food we eat. Glutathione is synthesized inside
the cells as required, from the building blocks supplied in the foods or
food supplements that we should eat. As a result, the cell retains direct
control of its chief defensive weapon. Nature obviously knows best.

Cellular GSH therefore plays a central role in defending mammalian bodies against such insults as infection, free radicals and potential carcinogens (foreign chemicals or xenobiotics). It is also known to function directly or indirectly in many important biological phenomena, including the synthesis of proteins and DNA, synthesis of prostaglandins and leukotrienes, amino acid transport, enzyme activity and metabolism. Table 5 is a convenient summary of the key functions of GSH.

Table 5.   Glutathione Functions

1.   Enhancing The Immune System
Your body's immune activity, involving unimpeded multiplication of lymphocytes and antibody production, requires mainte nance of normal levels of glutathione inside the lymphocytes.

2.   Antioxidant And Free Radical Scavenger
Glutathione plays a central protective role against the damag ing effects of bacteria, viruses, pollutants and free radicals.

3.   Regulator Of Other Antioxidants
Without *glutathione*, other important antioxidants such as vita mins C and E cannot do their job adequately to protect your body against disease.

4.   A Detoxifying Agent
Another major function of *glutathione* is the detoxification of foreign chemical compounds such as carcinogens and harmful metabolites.

Glutathione is a powerful and important detoxifier of mammalian cells and of the human body in particular. We are exposed to toxins on a daily basis: toxins in the food supply, in the water we drink and most certainly in the air we breathe. The level of intracellular GSH has a direct effect on the body's ability to neutralize and eliminate these toxins. It is not surprising that the highest levels of glutathione are found in the liver and in the kidneys, the two major organs involved in detoxification and elimination. Studies already demonstrate the effective role of GSH in counteracting the potential damage caused by autoemissions, cigarette smoke, radiation, sunburn, heavy metals like mercury and lead, and other environmental chemicals. It has been shown that glutathione neutralizes oxidation products, quenches reactive free radicals, and/or combines with enzyme systems to conjugate (or bind) with toxic substrates to facilitate their elimination from cells individually and from the body as a whole.

Glutathione not only acts as a principal antioxidant and detoxifier but it is a central player in the functioning of the immune system. It is a limiting factor in the proper activity of human lymphocytes. When the body is invaded by any pathogen or there is a change in tissue cells that spell trouble, lymphocytes multiply rapidly to mount a counter attack. This consumes oxygen, produces oxidative stress as described above and thereby taxes the available glutathione. Research indicates that elevated glutathione levels enable the system to be much more effective, and on the contrary, low levels weaken the immune system – as seen in AIDS patients, in the extreme case.

The multifunctional properties of glutathione become even more obvious by observing the wide variety of basic research areas addressed in the publications on the subject. These include enzyme mechanisms, biosynthesis of macromolecules, intermediate metabolism, drug metabolism, radiation, carcinogenesis, oxygen toxicity, transport, immune phenomena, endocrinology, environmental toxins, aging and much, much more. This is clearly a molecular focus for the twenty-first century.

SUPPLY AND DEMAND

Recall that glutathione is only synthesized inside the cell. Fig. 4 earlier showed a simplified reaction scheme. Although, in principle, the inflow of cysteine, glutamate and glycine into the cell could prove somewhat limiting under select circumstances, many observations have shown that cysteine availability is indeed *the* rate-limiting factor in GSH synthesis. Glycine and glutamate are readily available in typical North American diets, but cysteine is much harder to come by.

Many attempts have been made to enhance intracellular glutathione, but beside the use of whey protein concentrate, all other approaches have proved futile for a number of different reasons. The major attempts to date would include the following:

(i)   **Administration of glutathione (GSH) itself.** Attempts by oral, intravenous, intratracheal or intraperitoneal routes have no sustained effect.

Oral (by mouth):   GSH is available in fresh fruit, vegetables and meats, or may be made synthetically. But GSH is digested or broken down into its amino acid constituents and by themselves, those have no effect on raising intracellular GSH levels.

Intravenous (by needle): GSH has a very short half-life in the circulation.

Intratracheal(by aerosol inhalation): GSH would only affect the respiratory linings, briefly.

Intraperitoneal (by abdominal wall): GSH plasma levels rise but there is no increase in the tissues such as the liver, lung or lymphocytes.

(ii)   **Chemically altered glutathione.** Synthetic derivatives of glutathione such as mono – or di-esters can make effective delivery systems. Some increases in the levels of glutathione have been noted in specific tissues, but the widespread application is limited, particularly because of the harmful or even toxic products of metabolism, such as alcohol and acetaldehyde.

(iii)   **Amino Acid building blocks.** Oral supplementation with sulfur-containing amino acids such as cysteine and methionine, tend to be associated with toxicity. (This is especially so in premature infants, in alcoholics and after surgical stress). Cysteine itself, when consumed directly, is unstable in the bloodstream and as such, can be oxidized into potentially toxic byproducts including the lethal hydroxy radical. In any case, it does not cross the cell membrane effectively and that it must, if it is to affect glutathione systhesis. Clinically, animals fed oral cysteine show no positive response. The other sulfur-containing amino acid, methionine, can be converted into cysteine in the body when the liver is healthy, but it does have a tendency to also convert into homocysteine which is itself associated with increasing risk of heart disease.Cysteine is also readily metabolized.

(iv)   **Increasing protein intake**. Nutritional efficiency, as measured by the protein content of the diet, is unrelated per se to the level of glutathione inside the cells. Most commercial whey protein concentrates or casein prove ineffective in raising the lymphocyte GSH in laboratory animals and the effect is clearly not sustained. Obviously, these commercial dry whey isolates are prepared under routine conditions that *denature the essential but fragile proteins so as to destroy their bioavailability,* even though their food value remains. They may help to build *body mass* alright, but they are ineffective in *cell-defense.* However, decreased levels of glutathione have been found in many patient groups suffering from protein-energy malnutrition secondary to AIDS, cancer, alcoholism, chronic digestive disorder and burns. This is also a major complication for millions of children in developing countries who suffer from malnutrition (kwashiorkor) – a vicious cycle of disease.

(v)   **A few pharmaceutical drugs**:
N-ACETYL CYSTEINE(NAC) is commonly used as an antidote for acetaminophen (Tylenol™) poisoning and has also been looked at for treatment of HIV and AIDS patients. Orally, it has 10% bioavailability. By mouth or intravenously, the effect on glutathione levels is only temporary, and is best reserved for acute care in the emergency room or other critical areas. It has been used clinically to breakup mucus in lung diseases such as cystic fibrosis, chronic bronchitis, asthma and emphysema. Some oncologists have used it as an anti-cancer agent and to reduce the side effects of both chemo- and radiation therapy. At higher doses, side effects like gastro-intestinal upset and even cases of anaphylaxis, are not uncommon. Case reports of death

have even been documented. Yet, it is still the most commonly used method to raise GSH levels in clinical situations. Much has been learned about the important functions of GSH and the value of its modulation, from research using NAC as the available cysteine delivery system. It should have little relevance for the general population.

Another drug called **L-2-OXOTHIAZOLIDINE-4-CARBOXYLATE (O.T.C.),** a cysteine precursor as well, has also been used by mouth. It does provide some enhancement of glutathione levels. However, it is subject to feedback inhibition, and to nutritional regulation of glutathione synthesis. It therefore does not reliably produce a dramatic increase in tissue concentrations of glutathione.

(vi)   **Natural Products**

Lipoic Acid is a naturally occuring disulfide compound which is vital for converting glutathione (as well as other antioxidants like vitamins C and E and coenzyme Q10) back and forth from its oxidized to its reduced form. But it seems that GSH is the key player, the 'master antioxidant', and lipoic acid is one member of its supporting team. In fact, the critical enzyme glutathione-reductase has been shown to maintain lipoic acid in its reduced state. Lipoic acid has found clinical application and it does help restore glutathione when it is deficient.

Melatonin is a naturally occurring hormone derived from the amino acid tryptophan and the neurotransmitter serotonin. It has been shown to effectively raise glutathione levels in several tissues, especially including the brain. It too may be a member of the GSH-support cast.

Milk Thistle herb which we commented on in Chapter One, contains an active ingredient called silymarin which has been shown to also promote glutathione production. Traditionally, the plant has been used to treat a variety of liver disorders and in general is a 'detoxifier'.

All the above methods offer at best the interesting possibility for short-term or otherwise limited intervention. Their long term effectiveness in providing sustained increases in glutathione inside the cells has still not been confirmed and moreover, there is clearly potential toxicity.

Millions of lives have been saved by specific immunization vaccines, but there is **NO UNIVERSAL VACCINE** for the Immune System. **But Glutathione is** made by all cells for their own *internal* protection. This raises an interesting perspective. Is this nature's version of the same idea: **a single, effective agent of defense with ubiquitous efficacy against free radicals, oxygenated species and xenobiotics?** And now, thanks to the work of Dr. Gustavo Bounous and his colleagues, there is a safe, effective and convenient way to modulate the intracellular availability of this critical, defensive glutathione molecule.

The GSH antioxidant system is tightly regulated within the cell. Synthesis is increased on demand while over production is limited by feedback inhibition. In effect, each cell retains control of its own GSH status. Different conditions may coexist, with each one placing a demand for increased GSH. These might include:

- the production of oxygenated radicals inside the cell during immune response and cell proliferation;
- the metabolic consequences of strenuous muscle exercise such as seen in competitive (or at least serious) athletes post-exercise;
- the detoxification of foreign pollutants by ingestion or metabolism, or by inhalation or absorption through the skin; and/or
- the protection against radiation.

It is therefore conceivable that, during such severe challenges at least, there could be competition for inadequate GSH leading to functional deficiencies. In any case, the results Dr. Bounous and others observed in laboratory animals at least, clearly demonstrated the now understandable coincidence of the increasing tissue glutathione levels and the consistent beneficial effects of feeding with their unique whey protein concentrate.

But there is more. Even in disease states, glutathione exerts critical influence.

HUMAN TRIALS

Early studies had shown that the humoral immune response was significantly higher in *mice* fed a diet containing 20gm of whey protein concentrate per 100gm of diet than in *mice* fed formula diets of similar nutritional efficiency but where the "bioactive" whey was replaced by other semipurified food proteins. It was demonstrated that this immunoenhancing activity of the whey protein concentrate was related to greater production of splenic glutathione during the oxygen-requiring, antigen-driven clonal expansion of the lymphocyte pool. In addition, the *mice* fed the whey protein concentrate exhibited higher levels of tissue glutathione which was believed to account for observed antitumor effects and even favorable effects on natural aging.

These results were exciting and especially so when the pathophysiology seemed to be related to a common glutathione pathway. The literature was replete with studies on this fascinating intracellular tripeptide. It was known to be an amazing antioxidant, a free radical scavenger, a key co-factor in the influence of other antioxidants like vitamins C and E, and a major component of detoxifying enzyme systems in the liver. Now there was a handle on this ubiquitous cell defender. Indeed one could modulate glutathione with a simple dietary regime that was safe, effective and convenient.

Safety First

Yes, but that was all demonstrated in *mice*. Many a promising pharmaceutical product has been aborted in transition from laboratory bench to laboratory animals or from laboratory animals to human subjects. For a wide variety of reasons, a solution that works *in vitro* (in a test tube) may fail *in vivo* (in a live animal) or may be totally inapplicable for human application or treatment. Perhaps the human pathophysiology turns out to be different, or the side effects are awful, or the drug stability is inadequate, etc. So there could be big hurdles to climb in the shift from test tube, to laboratory animal to human beings.

But Bounous's whey protein concentrate was different from the outset. Here was a totally natural product wherein the common proteins of mother's breast milk were made available in concentrated form. What could be more natural? The effect was essentially to enhance glutathione production in cells by an intrinsic process which was itself regulated within *each* cell by feedback inhibition. What could be more safe? Elimination was by typical conversion of amino acid to urea for kidney excretion. What could be more predictable? This seemed from the beginning to be a naturally safe and predictable intervention.

So the question of safety of the whey protein concentrate seemed redundant although one could never be sure. One should never rush into human trials without due scientific consideration and review of all the available information. And protocol must be deliberately and systematically applied. Dr. Bounous believed in his nutritional innovation but before he rushed to human application, he wrestled with these considerations and more. He would only countenance doing the right thing in the right way and at the right time. He was a true scientist with deference for the clinicians.

AIDS

After Dr. Bounous and his colleagues published their research demonstrating the dramatic effects of the unique whey proteins and then elucidating the effective mechanism of glutathione modulation, a door was opened for further clinical inquiry. The first clinician to enter was Dr. Sylvain Baruchel, a researcher connected at that time to Montreal Children's Hospital. Dr. Bounous proposed a small pilot study, *to investigate the possible beneficial effect of Immunocal™ in symptom-free HIV-seropositive individuals.* After all, there is no better proof of efficacy in the immune system and no greater need in recent time, than the possible effect on patients with Human Immunodeficiency Virus (HIV) or Acquired Immune Deficiency Syndrome (AIDS). The syndrome is characterized by gross immunodeficiency, low T-helper cell blood content, increased oxidative stress and ... yes, systemic glutathione deficiency. Dr. Baruchel responded enthusiastically.

An AIDS Pilot Study

Immunocal™ was given orally to three male HIV-seropositive

individuals, ages 29-35. These patients took the product daily in a liquid of their choice for a period of 3 months. The daily intake of pure whey protein prescribed to the patients as Immunocal™ was increased step-wise. During the first 4 weeks, 8.4gm were prescribed daily; in the following 4 weeks, 19.6gm; and in the final 4-week period the dose was raised to 28gm (first week) and 39.2gm (last 3 weeks). Protein intake from other sources was reduced by corresponding amounts. In all these patients, there were no side effects and body weight increased progressively (from 2 to 7 kg); two of them reached ideal body weight. (The body weights of all three patients were low but stable for at least two months prior to the study.) Serum proteins, including albumin, remained unchanged and within normal range, indicating that protein replenishment per se was not likely the cause of the increased body weight.

The glutathione content of blood mononuclear cells was as expected, below normal values in all patients at the onset of the study. Over the 3-month period, however, glutathione levels increased and in one case, it rose by 70% to reach normal value. These objective changes were accompanied by a marked improvement of a subjective sense of well-being in all three patients. One patient, unduly concerned that the beneficial increase in body weight could hamper his preferred lean appearance, drastically reduced his Immunocal™ and total energy intake during the second period of study. During this time body weight increase was reduced and glutathione failed to rise. Three comparable patients on their usual standard diets over the same period, showed some weight loss and no change in their blood GSH mononuclear cell content.

The limited data indicated that whenever patients maintained their energy intake at pre-study levels but replaced a significant portion of the protein intake with Immunocal™, body weight increased and mononuclear cell glutathione increased.

This preliminary study published in 1993 clearly indicated the need for further clinical investigation on the effect of Immunocal™ in HIV-seropositive asymptomatic or symptomatic patients. **The whey proteins, by providing specific substrate containing cysteine for glutathione replenishment in the lymphocytes, could indeed represent an adjuvant at least to other forms of therapy.** These were remarkable results considering the alternatives available for HIV-seropositive individuals. This was even before widespread triple-drug therapy.

Children With AIDS

Dr. Baruchel became very interested in initiating a similar study in HIV-seropositive children. He led the Montreal group to conduct a Canadian clinical trial (Canadian HIV Trials Network) with Immunocal™ in children with AIDS and wasting syndrome. The major objective was *to evaluate the effect of oral supplementation with Immunocal™ on nutritional parameters and intracellular blood lymphocyte GSH concentration in such children.* This was an open single-arm pilot study of 6 months duration. Wasting syndrome and severe weight loss within the 6 months preceding entry into the study was an absolute criterion for entry.

In this protocol, Immunocal™ was administered twice a day as a powder diluted in water. In some patients, Immunocal™ was administered via nasogastric tube when necessary. The administered starting dose was based on 20% of the total daily protein requirement and was increased by 5% each month over 4 months to reach 35% of the total protein intake at the end of the study. The total duration of the study was 6 months.

The children were monitored regularly for their clinical response to the special diet. Weight, height, triceps skinfold and mid-arm muscle circumferences, CD4/CD8 counts, and peripheral lymphocyte GSH concentrations (measured by spetrophotometric assay) were measured monthly. Energy intake was assessed by the use of two independent 2-day food records with a 2-3 week period between the food records. Each food record included a weekday and a weekend, and the average of these records was calculated to reflect the daily nutritional intake. Out of 14 patients enrolled, 10 were evaluable. The ages of the patients ranged from 8 months to 15 years. The 10 patients studied were enrolled in four different centers across Canada: Montreal Children's Hospital (Dr. S. Baruchel), The Hospital For Sick Children Toronto (Dr. S. King), Children's Hospital For Eastern Ontario (Dr. U. Allen), and Centre Hospitalier Laval Quebec (Dr. F. Boucher). Of the 4 remaining patients, 2 lacked compliance after 2 months while the other 2 died of AIDS progressive disease within the first 2 months of entry into the study. None of the deaths was related to the tested product.

None of the patients experienced any major toxicity such as diarrhea or vomiting or manifestation of milk tolerance. One patient had to stop Immunocal™ transiently for minor digestive intolerance such as nausea and vomiting (<twice/day) at month 3 and was subsequently able to restart the treatment without any problem.

At the end of the study, all patients experienced a weight gain in the range of 3.2% to 22% from their starting weight. The mean weight gain for the group was 8.4% ± 5.7%. Recall that this was a reversal to the severe weight loss trend immediately prior to the study. On analysis of the mean percentage of Recommended Nutrient Intake (RNI) per month for all the patients, no correlation was found between the weight gain and any significant increase in the mean percentage of RNI, suggesting reduced catabolism rather than an anabolic effect of Immunocal™. Six of ten patients demonstrated an improvement in their anthropometric parameters such as triceps, skinfold or mid-arm muscle circumference independently of an increase in energy intake.

Two groups of patients were identified in terms of GSH (glutathione) modulation: responders and nonresponders. The responders were those who started the study with a low GSH level. The nonresponders were those who started with a normal GSH level. A positive correlation was found between increase in weight and increase in GSH. No changes were found in terms of blood lymphocyte CD4 cell count, but two patients exhibited an increase in the percentage of their CD8 cells and four patients showed a trend toward an increase in the number of NK cells.

In conclusion, this pilot study demonstrated that Immunocal™ is very well tolerated in children with AIDS and wasting syndrome and is associated with an amelioration of the nutritional status of the patient as reflected by weight and anthropometric parameters. Moreover, the GSH-promoting activity of Immunocal™ *in vivo* seemed to be validated in six out of ten patients.

(It is not surprising that the observed response was not 100 percent. This actually makes the reported data more credible. One should always beware of universal panaceas).

These results are consistent with a more recent discovery by Herzenberg and co-workers of the crucial importance of maintaining the GSH content of CD4 helper T-cells for the survival of HIV-infected patients. Hence, as was shown by Herzenberg in the area of survival, Baruchel's data substantiate the crucial correlation between GSH repletion and the patient's clinical improvement, i.e. cessation of wasting and/or increased body weight, unrelated to calorie intake.

In a joint research project with Dr. Mark Wainberg, Baruchel demonstrated further that Immunocal™, functioning as a cysteine delivery system, enhances GSH synthesis by mononuclear cells and inhibits HIV replication *in vitro*, as measured by reverse transcriptase activity in an infected cord mononucleated cell system. As well, Immunocal™ was found to inhibit the formation of syncitium between infected and non-infected cells and reduce apoptosis (cell death) of HIV-infected cells. The inhibition of syncitium formation occurred at the same concentration as the inhibition of HIV replication. These results were crucial to the understanding of the mechanism underlying the effect of Immunocal™ feeding in AIDS patients. The favorable clinical response could then be attributed to a direct anti-viral effect of raised GSH levels induced by some of the specific whey proteins.

In a further joint research project with Dr. René Olivier at the Pasteur Institute in Paris, Baruchel demonstrated that HIV-infected cells from AIDS patients when fed *in-vitro* with Immunocal™ would not die prematurely and would survive longer. These results generated major interest and were underlined by Dr. Luc Montagnier in the opening ceremony of the Tenth International AIDS Conference in Yokohama, Japan (1994) "as an important new line of research which should be expanded."

The new *in vitro* assay of GSH synthesis by mononucleated cells developed by Baruchel was also used to verify the bioactivity of different whey protein concentrates. Immunocal™ outperformed all the others. The same assay was also used for quality control of different future batches of Immunocal™. With these labile proteins, it is most important to safeguard consistent quality for reproducible results.

The results substantiated the proposal that normal GSH values in the mononucleated cells prevent HIV replication. On the other hand, HIV infection per se may directly affect GSH, as it decreases the activity of glucose– 6-phosphate dehydrogenase (G6PD), a key enzyme in the pathways that maintain GSH in its reduced state. Pulse administration of the cysteine derivative N-acetylcysteine (NAC) increased GSH blood level and survival in one study and plasma cysteine in another study. CD4+T-cell numbers did not, on the average, change significantly after N-acetylcysteine treatment.

Other case reports show that the administration of Immunocal™ can improve the clinical condition of HIV-infected patients even in the absence of anti-retroviral therapy. This favorable response may be associated with a decline of the plasma virus load, reflecting lowered virus production in the lymphoid tissue. However, at this time, *this form of dietary intervention should be viewed as complementary rather than an alternative to antiretroviral drug therapy.*

GSH Modulation And AIDS

Undenatured whey proteins and more specifically the cystine-rich thermolabile proteins represent an effective cysteine delivery system for the cellular synthesis of glutathione. The oral administration of these proteins (Immunocal™) induces a rapid replenishment of glutathione (GSH) in the lymphocyte during the GSH-depleting development of the immune response. Less hampered by oxiradicals, the lymphocyte can thus fully react with an optimal immune response to the antigenic stimulus. Similarly, the low GSH level in the lymphocytes of AIDS patients can be reconstituted to normal values by oral administration of Immunocal™.

The demonstration by Watanabe and others, that Immunocal™ increases GSH levels and inhibits the hepatitis B virus, supports the following hypothesis: the long incubation of the HIV virus until GSH levels drop in the lymphocyte hosting it, *suggests that the HIV virus cannot adapt by mutation to a normal GSH level as it would to external drugs*, because GSH is a natural component equally antagonistic to other viruses such as the viruses that cause hepatitis.

Immunocal™ might be viewed as a "natural" product with regard to its origin because it is derived from bovine milk and does not contain additives. However, its preparation involves the most advanced technology of micro-filtration, ultra-filtration and drying aimed at preserving the labile milk serum proteins in their natural form. That affords its *essential bioactivity*, acting as a cysteine delivery system for the cellular synthesis of glutathione.

Cellular glutathione (GSH) is a tightly self-regulated system because of the *feedback inhibition* of gamma-glutamylcysteine synthetase activity by the GSH level. However, when GSH is depleted, as in the lymphocytes of mice during the immune response or in the lymphocytes of AIDS patients, the cysteine delivery system in Immunocal™ produces a substantial increase in cellular GSH up to but not above normal values. Preliminary data in AIDS patients demonstrate that this is associated with major improvements in health.

These clinical data and the *in vitro* demonstration that Immunocal™ inhibits the HIV virus while increasing GSH synthesis, strongly suggest that *an antagonistic relation exists between the viruses and cellular GSH.*

Unlike specific antiretroviral drugs which may induce mutation hence resistance of the virus to therapy, the normalization of the lymphocyte glutathione levels and redox status through a cysteine delivery system represents *a totally different approach* by which the natural cellular defense system is boosted and against which the virus cannot apparently build up resistance by mutation.

CANCER

Within a few years after Dr. Bounous first discovered the quantitative immuno-enhancing property of his special whey protein concentrate, he and co-workers were daring enough to attempt, and surprisingly to prove, the anti-tumor effect at least in *mice* fed with a 20gm whey protein / 100gm diet. In particular, the chemically-induced colon tumors in these mice appeared to be similar to those found in humans insofar as the type of lesions and the chemotherapeutic response characteristics were concerned. Furthermore, the results with the whey protein concentrate feeding appeared to exert an inhibitory effect not only on the initiation of cancer, but also on the progression of tumors.

Similar results were also subsequently obtained in *rats* by Australian investigators. Dr. Graeme McIntosh and co-workers measured the input of different dietary protein sources on the incidence, burden and mass index of intestinal tumors induced by dimethylhydrazine in *rats*. They also found that whey proteins, in particular, offered considerable protection to the host against the chemically-induced tumors relative to other protein sources examined. Most recently, a study from Arkansas showed that diets formulated with special whey proteins provided significantly more protection than nutritionally equivalent casein or soy-based diets, against chemically-induced mammary cancer in multiparous female rats.

Again, it bears repetition – that reproducibility by other independent researchers in a true hallmark of good science. Nature is not capricious. Fundamentally, *science* exists and has utility only because of the true uniformity of *natural* causes. This confirmation of anti-tumor activity of special whey proteins in rats therefore validated the work of Dr. Bounous and his colleagues and provided encouragement to press on. This is important especially when one turns attention to a major disease process like *cancer in **humans***. That's what followed next.

Cancer Origins

Theories of the origin of cancer involve one or more of three kinds of molecular processes:

(i) free radical attack on key genes (oncogenes) in the DNA that cause on/off switches to initiate replication processes in renegade cell nuclei;

(ii) oxidative changes involving highly reactive oxygenated species that cause redox type phenomena which create havoc in cells; or

(iii) the poisoning effect of xenobiotics (foreign chemicals) that are toxic to normal cellular metabolism and biochemistry.

All these molecular effects are proposed to alter gene expression in one way or another. This leads then to mutations or changes inside the cells. If these conditions persist, the cells continue to malfunction and propagate the dire consequences.

Research on glutathione has elucidated the key role that this singular intracellular molecule plays in countering all three types of molecular processes just described above. **Glutathione is the cells' principal free radical scavenger and antioxidant, as well as a key player in the enzyme detoxification of carcinogens by conjugation.**

The search for ways to inhibit cancer cells without injuring normal cells has been based over the years on a vain effort to identify the metabolic parameters in which cancer cells are at variance with normal cells. One such function could very well be the all-important synthesis of cellular glutathione. Indeed, researchers found elevated intracellular glutathione levels in their cancer cells compared to normal cells, presumably related to their proliferative activity. More specifically, an *in vitro* assay showed that Bounous's special whey protein concentrate caused GSH *depletion and inhibition of proliferation of cells in a rat model of human mammary carcinoma.* The selectivity demonstrated by Baruchel in these experiments could be explained by the fact that GSH synthesis is negatively inhibited by its own synthesis and since, as mentioned earlier, baseline intracellular GSH is higher in tumor cells, it is easier to reach the level at which negative feedback inhibition occurs in this cellular system compared to a non-tumor cellular system. In addition, patients taking Immunocal™ exhibited substantial increases in NK-cell activity.

In any case, the dramatic anti-tumor effect that Dr. Bounous discovered in *mice* was crying out for an attempt at human application.

A Cancer Pilot Study

In testing a new approach to cancer treatment, patient selection and accrual are difficult issues. The selected patients must have a reasonable life expectancy, and must have measurable disease. They must not be denied available standard therapy and must understand the rationale of the proposed treatment in order to be able to sign an informed consent. Thus, only a small number of subjects could be selected for a pilot study and, for ethical reasons, a control group was not included.

A Phase I-II clinical trial was undertaken to test the effect of Immunocal™ in five patients with metastatic breast cancer, one with pancreatic cancer and another with metastatic adenocarcinoma to the liver of unknown primary. Under the circumstances, it proves difficult to enlist patients for this kind of innovative trial. It is not surprising that the few consenting patients prove more often than not, to be quite seriously ill. The inclusion criteria for the patients were as follows.

1. Histology (microscopic slides for cell type analysis and pathology) was available for review.

2. Measurable disease was present in soft tissues, lymph nodes, lungs, liver or bones.
3. No chemotherapy, radiotherapy or hormonal therapy had been given within three months of starting therapy with Immunocal™
4. Informed consent was obtained.
5. Life expectancy was at least six months.

For this small study, Drs. Bounous and Baruchel in Montreal collaborated with Drs. Renee Kennedy, George Konok and Timothy Lee at Dalhousie University and the Halifax Infirmary Hospital in Nova Scotia, Canada.

Immunocal™ was administered as a daily dose of 30 gram of powder dissolved in a liquid of the patient's choice. The patient's diet was assessed for the six months to rule out excessive protein intake which has been shown to potentially enhance tumor growth. Each patient had a full clinical assessment at the time of entry into the study and at three and six months after initiation of therapy. Relevant imaging studies were done at the same time intervals. They were also seen bi-weekly for the assessment of their general condition, weight, tolerance to and compliance with the Immunocal™ therapy. Complete blood counts, serum albumin, total protein and standard liver function tests were obtained. An aliquot of blood was drawn for lymphocyte isolation and measurement of intracellular glutathione.

Most of the patients could be characterized as "responders", or "non-responders" based on the correlation between their clinical course and their blood GSH levels. Six patients started with substantially elevated values compared to known normal values as well as a simultaneously performed normal control. Those who showed only a brief response had an initial drop in their lymphocyte GSH levels which corresponded to their clinical picture. However, as their disease progressed, the GSH levels began to rise, once again (patients 4-6). Those who had a favourable, and more protracted clinical response to Immunocal™, had noticeable and sustained drops in their GSH levels (patients 1,3). In some patients, positive clinical results were associated with increased haemoglobin (patients 1-3) and peripheral blood lymphocytes (patients 1,3) and normalization of platelet counts (patients 1,5), all of which are indirect measures of disease regression.

An interesting phenomenon was observed in that every patient experienced a period of improved sense of well-being, which while difficult to quantify, was appreciable in all patients. In some, it led to a perceived improvement in the quality of life for at least a short duration, and some patients were able to perform activities they could not previously. The number in the study was too small to draw firm conclusions from this, especially without matched controls, but *the results were encouraging.*

Case Reports

In the absence of large-scale clinical trials at the present time, it is further encouraging to find a number of credible Case Reports that show the effect of the same specifically prepared whey protein concentrate (Immunocal™) on urogenital cancers in particular. These have been recently presented by Dr. Bounous and is currently (at the time of writing) *in press* for academic publication. They include clinical submissions from seven (7) different medical centers.

As we discussed back in Chapter Three, case reports are only a scientific version of anecdotal experience which provides adequate documentation. It is improper to draw any major conclusions from these but it is clearly encouraging when clinicians in several different centers all report positive results for any particular novel intervention in patients with well-characterized illness. Further research on a larger population should certainly be conducted in order to validate these limited findings. That poses major demands and challenges for clinicians but it is definitely the way forward as we seek to understand the dramatic role of glutathione modulation by cysteine precursors found in this unique whey protein concentrate – a derivative from nature's goldmine.

Adjuvant Therapy

A major problem in the use of chemotherapeutic agents in cancer treatment is the protection offered by the defense mechanisms of the tumor cells. An important element of protection is represented by glutathione which is an effective detoxification agent, relatively abundant in tumor cells. Immunocal™ favorably influences the GSH synthesis in normal cells. Hence, this nutritional supplement while exerting an inhibitory effect per se on cancer cell GSH and replication, could also be viewed as an adjunct to chemotherapy. Lower GSH levels could in fact, render cancer cells more vulnerable to chemotherapeutic agents. The validity of this assumption is substantiated by the observation of Hercbergs and others, that cancer patients are more likely to respond to chemotherapy if their erythrocyte GSH, (and by inference tumor GSH), concentrations are low.

Given the technical and ethical difficulties in monitoring tumor tissue GSH during cancer treatment, peripheral blood lympocyte GSH levels were taken in the pilot study described above, as a reflection of those in tumor cells. This assumption is substantiated by a previous study of a large series of cancer patients in whom erythrocyte GSH concentration was found to reflect tumor cell GSH on the basis of differential tumor responses to chemotherapy.

In view of the advantages of reduced intracellular levels of GSH in tumor cells and increased levels in the normal cells of the host, it seems noteworthy to have found in the patients who performed well on Immunocal™, the highest levels of initial lymphocyte GSH. These values fell into normal range soon after Immunocal™ was initiated and remained so through the six months of treatment. In the patients exhibiting disease progression, the GSH levels tended to rise. It is felt that the high lymphocyte levels of GSH occur as a result of a leaching effect from the tumor to the lymphocytes. These lymphocyte values are therefore felt to be an indirect measure of tumor levels, as were the erythrocytes in the previously quoted study by Hercbergs and coworkers.

This preliminary study, indicated at least that *this newly discovered property of whey proteins may be a promising adjunct in the nutritional management of cancer patients about to undergo chemotherapy.* Selective depletion of tumor GSH may in fact render the malignant cells more vulnerable to the action of chemotherapeutic agents.

RE-THINKING MEDICINE

Just pause for a minute and reflect on what is being discussed in this chapter. Think of how the body defends itself. At the most fundamental level of the immune system, each cell has its own protective strategy to resist the biochemical changes that threaten its own survival. Surely it has a sophisticated membrane that defines its integrity and limits the unwanted intrusion from the external environment. It also has its own genetic machinery to dictate what happens internally. But it is at risk of premature oxidation, of free radical damage, of chemical poisoning by invading toxins, and of the devastating influences of other microbes like viruses and bacteria that are engaged in a war of survival. A critical strategy for the cell in its own defense, is to produce glutathione *internally* on demand, to serve as 'master antioxidant', free radical scavenger, detoxifier and a special boost to critical fighting cells of the immune system. That's *nature* at work.

Now, think again of the discovery of Dr. Bounous and his colleagues. Using as natural a product as unique whey protein concentrate, they find a safe, effective and convenient way to modulate glutathione production inside human cells. It is an intervention that imitates what *nature* already does in the provision of the same proteins in mother's breast milk for the defense of the vulnerable newborn baby. In breast milk, it is essentially prophylaxis – a pro-active provision to prevent disease. The technology to isolate the same bioactive proteins from a common source and deliver a concentrate that can up-regulate intracellular glutathione production *in vivo* is good *science* at work.

Who would imagine that such an intervention would have the effects we have noted above in patients with major illnesses like AIDS or cancer. These are very complex diseases as we have found out. After most of the best minds in science and medicine have made major concerted research efforts on both of these conditions around the world, we are still a long way from curing either of these diseases. Glutathione modulation is certainly not a cure, but the results to date are encouraging and support the contention that there is some value in this *complementary* approach to both disease prevention and management for patients at risk of either condition.

Furthermore, now that we have grasped the importance of cell-defense per se, and the role of glutathione as a critical defensive player; and now that we have a safe, effective and convenient way to modulate intracellular glutathione levels – we ought to rethink and inquire into the possible impact of this intervention in primary prevention and in many pathological states that clinicians seek to manage on a daily basis. In a word, we need to re-think modern medicine, at least from this perspective, as we search for new prospects and directions for health care.

In a new book on *"Glutathione – Your body's most powerful healing agent"*, Dr. Jimmy Gutman (with Stephen Schettini) has reviewed the abundant literature on GSH that underscores its relevance to a wide variety of physiological processes and clinical conditions. The research data indicates that glutathione level is a valuable clinical indicator and often a predictor of many conditions in both health and disease. We will summarize its role in just a few select areas of current medical interest.

Cardiovascular Disease

Heart disease and stroke are the leading cause of death in North America at the turn of this new century. The common pathological process is atherosclerosis or hardening of the arteries. There is now good scientific evidence that glutathione is involved in both the prevention and prognosis of these conditions.

Oxidative stress is a key factor in the build up of *bad LDL cholesterol* and in the early plaque formation in the arterial lumen. It leads to lipid peroxidation and free radical formation, which some cardiologists believe could be minimized by use of antioxidants. It has been suggested that even in an acute setting, the use of antioxidant therapy prior to procedures such as thrombolysis, angioplasty or coronary bypass, may help to reduce possible complications. Other cardiologists may be skeptical but it is interesting to note that a recent poll of cardiologists published in the American Journal of Cardiology, found that as many as 44% of these specialists who responded, themselves take antioxidants.

It has been shown that the decreasing levels of glutathione with age contribute to the formation of *atherosclerosis*. Two of the biochemical markers for cardiovascular risk – namely, lipoprotein-A and homocysteine – have both been shown to decrease substantially when glutathione levels were raised by the application of the drug, N-acetyl cysteine (NAC). When the GSH levels in the red blood cells of some heart attack victims were measured, there was evidence of glutathione depletion. That was probably a consequence of the major event rather than a direct cause.

When bypass surgery or thrombolytic drugs are used to restore circulation and oxygen supply to tissues after a blood clot, there is an increased oxidative stress which can cause further damage. This *reperfusion injury* requires adequate antioxidants to minimize its effect. Cardiologists have measured GSH depletion after cardiac ischemia, and shown that administration of NAC can combat this.

Increased levels of GSH are known to improve the reduction of overall cholesterol by raising the activity of the enzyme cholesterol hydroxylase. Even selenium which is known to correlate well with levels of good cholesterol, seems to exert its influence in the formation of another enzyme, glutathione peroxidase. In the general circulation, there is yet a role for glutathione in maintaining smooth muscle tone in the walls of the vessels, and the shifts and balances in important clotting variables such as prostaglandins, leukotrienes, thromboxanes and clotting factors.

In the brain, studies in animals have shown that when the levels of glutathione were artificially lowered, they suffered significantly more brain damage after a stroke. Other neurosurgeons reported that depleting glutathione also caused the constriction of some critical arteries supplying those areas starved of oxygen.

There is obviously much more work to be done in this area, but it is time for many more cardiologists to inquire further into the surprising role and opportunity with glutathione in cardiovascular disease.

Respiratory Illness

Every medical student quickly learns the A, B, C, of patient care: A-Airway, B-Breathing and C-Circulation. That's the order of importance. After all, continuous oxygen supply is indispensable to life – even moreso than water and food. But the same process of respiration creates oxidative stress locally in the lungs and other respiratory tissue and the importance of glutathione in this system is clearly apparent. The huge quantities of oxidation products must be neutralized. Add to that the airborne pollutants, especially cigarette smoke, and common inhaled infectious agents and the need is further exaggerated. Fortunately, the lining of the respiratory tree can absorb glutathione directly. Other organs can only synthesize GSH from precursors available in the diet or as drugs. Clinically, topical forms of GSH and NAC have been developed as aerosols/sprays for treatment of a number of respiratory diseases. Oral and intravenous GSH precursors are now being actively studied in this regard, even in acute settings such as intensive care units.

There are a large number of different respiratory diseases but there is often a common inflammatory response associated with further oxidative stress. Glutathione is then a fairly common antedote for both obstructive and restrictive conditions, so that modulating GSH levels is then a most appropriate intervention.

Asthma is one of the most common causes of absenteeism and hospitalization in children in school and is fairly prevalent even in adults. The clinical condition varies widely but several studies have shown that glutathione and glutathione peroxidase are important in the onset and progression of asthma. There is a direct correspondence between low levels of GSH (in red and white blood cells, serum platelets and lung fluid) and the severity of asthma attack. Some physicians have used GSH precursors in treatment, especially to break up thick secretions and NAC has proved a useful adjuvant to inhaled bronchodilators in one double-blind study.

Patients with *chronic obstructive pulmonary disease* (COPD) – including both chronic bronchitis and emphysena – can have major secondary complications. NAC has been shown to produce improvements in symptoms and pulmonary function in a large open study of over 2000 COPD patients. Smoking is the principal cause of COPD and several other diseases. The smoke is loaded with free radicals and toxins, which trigger lung inflammation – all sources of oxidative stress. NAC and inhaled GSH are being studied as adjuvant therapy for these COPD cases too. Professor Lands and colleagues from McGill University recently published a Case Report in *Chest* of a 40 year old patient with worsening COPD, but responsive to corticosteroids, and with low (whole blood) glutathione levels. Following one month of supplementation with Immunocal™, GSH levels increased, but more importantly, pulmonary function significantly and dramatically increased and continued to remain so on this therapy alone. Some French researchers reported a correlation between a specific GSH enzyme and smokers who develop moderate and severe bronchitis.

Acute respiratory distress syndrome (ARDS) is an even more acute, life-threatening condition associated often with respiratory failure. These patients have extremely high levels of oxidative stress with large amounts of free oxygen radicals, hydrogen peroxide and other lethal oxygen species. Not surprising, clinical trials show that with intravenous NAC (and also OTZ, or pro-cysteine), there is increased oxygen delivery, improved elasticity (compliance) in the lung, reduced edema and overall improvement in pulmonary function.

For a variety of reasons, the lung tissue itself can become scarred and stiff giving rise to difficulty in clearing secretions and in gas exchange. Oxidative stress is an important factor in the causes and conditions of such *pulmonary fibrosis*. Both NAC and aerosol GSH have proven valuable in the management of these patients, resulting again in improved pulmonary function. GSH may indeed slow the progress of pulmonary fibrosis.

One respiratory condition that cannot be overlooked is *cystic fibrosis*. It is an inherited disease affecting some 30,000 North Americans who live typically to early adult life. They have serious difficulty in clearing secretions of all kinds but become trapped in a cycle of inflammation and infection. GSH is noticeably depleted in all the intense oxidative stress. NAC aerosols have been used for some time to break up mucus plugs (as in the case of other obstructive lung diseases) but more recently, attention has been given to oral glutathione precursors such as Immunocal™ in comprehensive management.

Clearly, the widespread importance of glutathione in pulmonary disease demands more concerted efforts to understand the clinical implications of GSH modulation. We can expect increasing application of this type of intervention in all types of respiratory problems over the next few years.

Gastrointestinal Disorders

Just as the airways and lungs provide direct interaction with the air we breathe, so the digestive tract is the direct interface with the food we eat and fluids we drink. The process of digestion itself produces metabolites and general waste that must be eliminated expeditiously before toxicity, inflammation and infection overwhelm the natural defense. Speaking of defense, glutathione plays a crucial role again in protecting the entire digestive mucosa from mouth to anus.

In *the stomach*, glutathione offers protection against oxidative stress, detoxifies potentially harmful and even carcinogenic substances and mediates the various immune mechanisms to afford a more effective immune response. Alcohol induces an elevation of GSH at low to moderate levels, and causes damage at higher levels when the system is overwhelmed. The gastric side-effects of common anti-inflammatory drugs are significantly reduced when GSH or cysteine is ingested at the same time. Chronic inflammation and the infectious bacteria *Heliobacter Pylori* cause increases in free radical damage and GSH turnover in the mucosa. Decreasing GSH and GSH-dependent enzymes correlate with increase in peptic and duodenal ulcers. Using NAC as adjuvant to conventional ulcer treatment (antibiotics, H2 –blockers, mucosal barriers and motility agents) has shown good results. Similarly, low GSH levels also correlate with the development of stomach cancer.

The pancreas produces digestive enzymes and important hormones (insulin, glucagon) and is also subject to oxidative stress. Glutathione depletion is found in all early stages of pancreatitis and supplementation with GSH and GSH precursors can protect the pancreas from auto-digestive enzymes and external toxins like alcohol, and then help to prevent the subsequent damage to other tissues if pancreatitis progresses.

The two major inflammatory diseases of the bowel, *ulcerative colitis and Crohn's disease*, show consistent evidence of severe oxidative stress. The extent of inflammation correlates directly with the degree of oxidative damage. Again, there is significant depletion of glutathione and related enzymes. The latter suggests that this may be a contributing cause and not just a consequence of the inflammation. In any case, antioxidant therapy has emerged as a complementary approach to the more standard treatment (aminosalicylate drugs and steroids, plus or minus surgery). With Crohn's especially, nutrient absorption can be a problem and GSH levels are generally depleted throughout the body. Just as aerosols have effectively delivered glutathione and its precursors for direct absorption in the respiratory tree, so ingestion of glutathione raises GSH levels in the mucosa by direct contact and provides some local protection.

Inflammation of *the liver* is caused mainly by alcohol (and other toxins) or virus (hepatitis A, B or C) infection. The extent of liver inflammation determines how well the liver can function. Among the many critical functions, detoxification in the liver is life saving. Glu-tathione is the most abundant antioxidant and detoxifier, collaborating with other critical enzymes. It has been known for a long time that liver damage invariably depletes GSH which causes more dysfunction, and the cycle continues. The classic medical application of the GSH-en-hancing (precursor) drug N-acetylcysteine (NAC) is the (intravenous) drug of choice for acute overdose of hepatotoxic pharmaceutical drugs, especially common acetaminophen (Tylenol™ etc). This raises GSH levels rapidly and neutralizes the toxic metabolites from the overdose. But in both toxic and viral hepatitis it is generally important to raise glutathione levels to help restore normal liver function. Both the immu-nological parameters and the liver function abnormalities in hepatitis B patients have been improved during and even after treatment with Immunocal™, the same unique whey protein concentrate that Dr. Bounous found to increase intracellular glutathione. NAC has also been demonstrated as a useful adjuvant to interferon treatment in hepatitis C patients.

Again, it is clear that oxidative stress is a ubiquitous factor in diseases of the gastrointestinal tract. Glutathione in the mucosa and other tissues is central to both protective and reactive strategy in these associated conditions. Modulation of glutathione provides an increas-ingly useful intervention and offers further hope for the future.

Neurodegenerative Disease

As the population ages, there is a corresponding interest in neurodegenerative diseases which can dramatically affect the quality of life in later years. Although Parkinson's disease and Alzheimers dis-ease are considered diseases of old age, an estimated half of the 3 mil-lion Parkinson patients are believed to have had symptoms by age 40, whereas 5-10% of all adults over age 65 are affected by Alzeheimer's. In both cases, there is a recognized role of oxidative stress.

The classic symptoms of *Parkinsons* – T.R.A.P. for tremor, rigidity, akinesia and postural disturbance – derive from decreasing dopamine production from nerve cells in a particular part of the mid-brain. It is clearly a multi-factoral condition involving genetics, medi-cations, viruses, pesticides, repetitive head trauma, carbon monoxide, manganese, cyanide and more. Typical treatment has involved replacing dopamine and minimizing the side effects. A promising new drug called selegiline may (amongst other things) increase GSH activity.

The associated extensive oxidative stress and circulatory free radicals are consistent with the GSH depletion in the brain tissues. Those levels decrease up to 40% in the early stages and by the late stages they fall to a mere 2% of normal. Research has shown that elevated GSH levels slow brain tissue damage, even more effectively than other anti-oxidants like vitamins C and E. The effects are seen in both early and later stages of the disease and the improvement observed dissipates within months after the GSH modulation is stopped.

Clearly, the early results are promising for Parkinson's patients and GSH modulation promises to be a useful complement to standard drug therapy and conventional care.

Alzheimer's disease is a progressive, degenerative illness, characterized in life by deteriorating brain function (dementia, memory loss, mood changes, confusion and disorientation etc.) and at post-mortem by pathological tissue signs (neurofibrillary tangles and plaques). There is global neurodegeneration with shrinkage of the brain as a whole. It is believed to involve certain proteins (ApoE is the latest suspect) reacting with heavy metals like aluminum and mercury, as well as iron, zinc and calcium.

Post-mortem studies on Alzheimer patients show changes in GSH and GSH peroxidase levels as well as increased lipid peroxide. Glutathione levels are diminished in the hippocampus, the area of the brain responsible for short-term memory, as well as in the cerebral cortex involved in higher intellectual functioning. Most particularly, the probable role for GSH in the elimination and detoxification of heavy metals is inviting, especially since benefits have already been observed with more traditional chelating agents.

The exact pathogenesis of Alzheimer's is not yet clear but it is certain that oxidative stress and free radical damage are involved as a cause or consequence of the crucial reactions of proteins with heavy metals. Clearly more research is warranted to further assess the effects of glutathione modulation in these neurodegenerative pathologies.

Autoimmune Disease

We briefly discussed autoimmunity in Chapter Four when we

detailed some of the known science of the immune system. Having seen the importance of glutathione in the immune response it would not be surprising to find a role for GSH in autoimmune disease. It is helpful to note that although glutathione enhances the immune response, it does not follow that it would exaggerate the unwanted aspects of autoimmuity . In fact autoimmuity, we pointed out earlier, is a failure in target recognition on the one hand, and/or a failure in the balanced regulatory control which should suppress the unwanted immune response to 'self' antigen. Let's look at three different types of autoimmune disease: rheumatoid arthritis, multiple sclerosis and diabetes.

In *rheumatoid arthritis* (RA), several joints show symptoms of chronic inflammation which result from oxidation and free radical damage. It is believed that the local B-cells are overactive and T-cells (especially T-suppression cells) are ineffective. Evidence shows that the GSH content of T-cells in the rheumatoid joints is lower than that in the systemic T-cells of the same RA patients. Administration of NAC to raise GSH levels in these tissues has yielded definite improvement in the inflammatory changes at the cellular level.

The causes of *multiple sclerosis* (MS) have been debated for years but at least to most immunologists, MS is most likely an autoimmune disorder destroying the myelin sheath that insulates and protects nerve fibers. It is a neurodegenerative disorder like Alzheimer's or Parkinson's and here again, studies do suggest that oxygen-derived free radicals and inadequate antioxidant defenses play some important role in the pathogenesis. The myelin sheaths are comprised of fatty lipids vulnerable to peroxidation. The actual diseased nerve tissues show damage by cytokines which are known to generate free radicals in abundance. Pre-treating these tissues with NAC to raise GSH levels protected them from demyelination and depleting GSH made it worse. Clinically, the levels of oxidative stress correlates with the severity of the MS attack (comparable to what we noted about asthma). One research group in fact postulated that macrophages attack myelin and release enzymes, peroxides etc. to cause extensive oxidative stress. That consumes GSH and when the cerebrospinal fluid is examined in MS patients, GSH levels are indeed consistently low. In the MS nerve plaques themselves, GSH is almost absent. Low selenium levels also correlate with MS occurrence and this trace mineral is known as an essential atom in GSH peroxidase, again consistent with the GSH role. In the light of all this, clearly one should address MS, not only with supportive care and traditional but inadequate immunosuppression therapy, but we need attempts to reduce oxidative damage, particularly by elevating glutathione levels. That's a new frontier for an old debilitating illness that unfortunately, affects many younger people.

The third autoimmune disease we will comment on is *diabetes*. More specifically in Type 1 or juvenile-onset diabetes the islet cells of the pancreas that make insulin are destroyed and insulin therapy becomes mandatory. There is good evidence of autoimmunity contributing to this disease. For example, there is an association with a specific MHC (HLA) marker, just as for multiple sclerosis or adult rheumatoid arthritis. The possible effect of oxidative stress, and therefore of GSH in protecting the islet cells from autoimmune attack, has not yet been elucidated. However, the complications that follow both Type I and Type II (adult-onset) diabetes have definite involvement of oxidative stress and an increased need for a heightened immune system, given the increased vulnerability to infection and vascular compromise. The blood and tissues of diabetics are characteristically low in GSH and the low GSH correlates directly with increased complications of diabetes.

Much research still needs to be done in this area but a general point should be made. Often, doctors target treatment for specific disease indications. However, **since oxidative stress is so widespread either as a contributing cause or an exacerbating consequence of many illnesses, and too, since the immune response is a common defensive strategy almost inevitably, then the practice of glutathione modulation to affect both of these areas makes consummate sense in almost any kind of clinical condition.** It is more a strategy to be deployed than a weapon to be fired – that necessitates a re-thinking of medicine too.

The Reproductive Spectrum

Finally, we should consider issues that span the entire reproductive spectrum from conception and gestation, to delivery and lactation. After all, this is a major fraction of all we try to do in medicine and literally dictates the hope for the future of young children and the world.

Not much has been done in the area of *infertility* and glutathione.

But as we re-think medicine from this perspective, questions arise concerning the role of oxidative stress in the ovary where germ cells ('eggs') survive for years and only come to individual maturation for release each month during a woman's reproductive years. And then there is the sperm, cradled by the millions in a fluid matrix for the strongest and quickest to triumph by natural selection. Is GSH a discriminating factor? Then, when sperm meets egg and they get their act together, is oxidation or pre-mature oxidation relevant? Are there any immune influences? Recall that the scientific method begins with asking the right questions.

In any case, some women the world over, conceive each day by the awesome miracle of nature. During months of gestation, both mother and fetus are challenged continuously and many things can go wrong. We do know that glutathione is implicated in a number of these conditions in pregnancy. We know that hypertensive pregnant mothers have consistently low GSH levels, which accounts for some of the important clinical observations. In *pre-eclampsia*, hypertension is accompanied by protein in the urine and swelling due to water accumulation in the hands, feet and face. Research shows a correlation between the severity of pre-eclampsia with cell fragility and the level of GSH-oxidation. In a bold attempt, the symptoms have been controlled in a test-group of pre-eclampsia patients (unresponsive to traditional therapy) with S-nitroso -glutathione.

Gestational diabetes is a further potential complication in pregnancy, leading sometimes to malformations and developmental problems if not managed well. Oxidative damage to cells is again important and GSH status is a good marker. NAC has proven to be protective in embryo tissue cultures. In the absence of diabetes, GSH levels are very high in the embryo's conceptual tissue. This is obviously and strategically protective. However, those levels can also be depleted by toxins, especially by alcohol and tobacco. The placenta itself is rich in GSH and as such neutralizes potential toxins to protect the fetus. In the laboratory, NAC reduces the toxic effects of xenobiotics like mercury on congenital abnormalities and even death.

Immediately after birth, the neonate must breathe on its own. Insufficient oxygen (*hypoxia*) is not uncommon and that can cause lipid peroxidation. As we have seen, glutathione is critical in all kinds of oxidative stress. In these circumstances, GSH stimulates production of the body's energy currency we call ATP, which again is anti-hypoxic. Classic treatment of hypoxia calls for oxygen therapy which can damage the eyes and have other side effects. Sustained levels of glutathione are again protective and furthermore, oxygen-induced lung injury has been reduced in mammals with GSH supplementation.

The final step in reproduction is that of *breast-feeding*, which brings us right back to what triggered this whole re-thinking process. We made the case for breast-feeding back in Chapter Two. Here it is important to note that human milk has this unique characteristic. It has the lowest proportion of proteins among mammals but a much higher whey to casein ratio. Those whey proteins are lactoglobulin, alpha-lactalbumin, serum albumin and lactoferrin. As we have seen in the last chapter – they contain high concentrations of the important glutathione precursor as cysteine and cystine (dimer).

That is *nature's* way of modulating glutathione for the vulnerable newborn. The *scientific* way is to carefully isolate these bioactive proteins from *cow's* milk (fortunately) and make them available to adults who also can benefit, as we have just seen, from increasing intracellular glutathione to do all that we now know it does and more.

Just consider again the spectrum of clinical conditions that we have commented on and briefly stated some of the key research results and the work in progress. We have gone from AIDS and cancer, to cardiovascular disease; to respiratory and gastrointestinal problems; then to neurodegenerative illness and autoimmune conditions; and finally, to issues of pregnancy and childbirth. One common thread has emerged. There is a ubiquitous demand on glutathione as the cells' key antioxidant and free radical scavenger (counteracting prevalent oxidative stress; as the key player in detoxification (and protection against xenobiotics); and as a major influence on the immune response (enabling the effective clonal expansion and the efficiency of critical immune cells). Now to gain a new safe, effective and convenient handle to modulate this same intracellular glutathione with unique whey protein concentrate similar to breast milk proteins – **That is a consummation of *nature* and *science*!** Thanks to nature's goldmine, it should help to detonate the glutathione revolution.

Healthy Adults

One further comment about re-thinking medicine. Already the public is re-thinking the traditional approach to the general practice of medicine, especially with its focus on diagnosis and therapeutics. In this they are ahead of the medical profession. They seem oblivious to all that doctors do in terms of prevention: immunizations, screening, public health programs etc. They want proactive guidance on daily living. So they turn to alternative practitioners for lifestyle advice and hands-on health intervention strategies. But good healthcare choices will inevitably demand a merger of these two streams. Empowering cells to defend themselves by the safe, effective and convenient route of glutathione modulation is a definite step in the right direction that the patient can take, with or without the advice of either traditional doctor or alternative practitioner. With such a well-documented rationale, both professionals and patient can work together in a new strategy of health promotion through enhanced self-defense. It's the best of prevention through basic self-help.

Prevention must be the important concern for all normal healthy adults. Even in the absence of clinical signs of illness or disease, glutathione is still at work. But the question arises: *Can supplementation with glutathione precursors lead to up-regulation or increase in tissue glutathione levels for the average healthy person?*

In a recent double-blind clinical study, the effect of supplementation with Immunocal™ on glutathione (GSH) levels and muscular performance in normal adults was observed by Dr. Larry Lands and co-workers. Since oxidative stress contributes to muscular fatigue and GSH is the major intracellular anti-oxidant, they hypothesized that supplementation to modulate GSH should enhance performance.

Twenty healthy young adults (10 males) were studied pre- and 3 months post-supplementation with either Immunocal™ (10 gm twice per day) or casein placebo. There were no initial baseline differences between the two groups (i.e. in age, height, weight, % ideal weight, Peak Power or 30-sec Work Capacity). One placebo subject dropped out, and one Immunocal subject's follow-up results were technically unacceptable. Lymphocyte GSH was used as a marker of tissue GSH. Muscular performance was assessed by whole leg isokinetic cycle testing, measuring Peak Power and 30-sec Work Capacity.

What were the findings?

(i.)   Lymphocyte GSH increased significantly in the Immunocal™ group (37.8±12.47%, p<0.03) with no change in the placebo group (0.9±9.6%).

(ii.)   Both Peak Power (mean rise 13±3.5%, p<0.02) and 30-sec Work Capacity (13±3.7%, p<0.03) increased significantly in the Immunocal™ group, with no significant change in the placebo group.

These results have clear implications.

Since normal healthy adults show such marked increases in glutathione levels when supplementary Immunocal™ is used, this self-regulated protective system (with its own feedback inhibition) may be operating below its optimum level, not only in persons with disease, but also in normal, healthy individuals.

The significant increase in physical performance observed also supports the use of such a well-tolerated whey-based cysteine donor to augment muscular performance. Other indices of well-being and fitness which are influenced by ongoing oxidative stress, may also be benefited by the same glutathione modulation.

As the major clinical indications for Immunocal™ continue to be investigated in the various types of studies just mentioned, there is therefore a need to remain focused on the important role of glutathione and hence Immunocal™, in primary disease prevention and wellness. After all, the key function of the immune system is to be pro-active. It seeks to be constantly on the alert to detect the enemy and mount a swift and effective defense in the pre-morbid condition. It is still worth repetition that 'an ounce of prevention is worth more than a pound of cure.'

We have clearly seen in the past three chapters, the value of pro-active intervention through glutathione modulation and its implications in terms of physical health and even areas of disease management. But it is obvious that health and wellness extends beyond the body to the state of the mind and therefore we must address areas of mental health. However, our methods should remain the same. We must look to *science* for understanding of the *nature* of mental processes and perhaps we might find another handle to exploit some other rich provision in nature's goldmine. In the next chapter, we will review the basic science of mental health and then we will go exploring in a subsequent chapter, in search of another revolutionary nugget.

PART
3

CALMING THE MIND

Chapter Seven

THE SCIENCE OF MENTAL HEALTH
Healthy body, healthy mind

The health-care practices that depart from the limited principles of orthodox medical care are described in a variety of ways, depending on what type of philosophy one wishes to emphasize. Those who promote *Traditional* remedies (like acupuncture for example) place the focus on the longevity of ancient healing arts. The advocates of *Alternative* medicine (such as naturopathy), emphasize the right of the individual patient to choose their own modality of health care. Promoters of *Holistic* or *Wholistic* medicine (not unlike Ayurvedic medicine) emphasize the body as an integral unit, with body, mind and spirit united in the 'whole' person. Practitioners of *Natural* therapies (like herbalism) draw attention to nature as the most safe and responsible source, in contrast to human technology and innovation. And finally, the proponents of *Complementary* medicine insist on the wise combination of both orthodox and unorthodox approaches to healthcare.

But whatever approach this contemporary movement takes, there are at least two unifying themes that remain consistent.

The first of these recurring themes is a claim to **strengthen the immune system**, whatever that means in the given context. Somehow, the unorthodox intervention is supposed to strengthen and enhance the body's innate capacity to defend itself and thus promote and maintain good health and healing, at least as best it can. We have noted earlier that responsibility and good science demands that whatever we do, we must concur with the known science of the immune system which we briefly reviewed in Chapter Four. The immune system is not an abstraction or some generalized ethereal force of nature at work in self-defense. It is a real elaborate, coordinated and measurable system of molecular parameters with defined structure and function. We now have verifiable data and some fair understanding of how the system works, so that any assertion that some intervention 'strengthens' or 'balances' the immune system should be elaborated in the context of that existing knowledge about the immune system. Anything less would fall into the category of folklore or fantasy.

The second common thread amongst the unorthodox approaches to healthcare is the assertion of the mind – body continuum and therefore the emphasis on individual perception, anecdotal experience and emotional well-being. It is as if the orthodox mantra 'above all, do no harm' has been translated **'no matter what, let them feel good'**. So much so, that the value of any healthcare protocol is often evaluated and promoted by the unorthodox in terms of personal testimonials and mental health influences.

This brings us to the very important area of health that relates to the psychological and behavioral aspects of wholeness and wellness – from the molecular events in the brain and central nervous system, to the social phenomena that define culture and civilization as a whole. In a word, we now turn attention to mental health.

The first *U.S. Surgeon General's Report on Mental Health* has just been published. It follows on the 1999 White House Conference on Mental Health. The formidable task was undertaken by two federal agencies – The Substance Abuse and Mental Health Services Administration (SAMHSA) and the National Institutes of Health (NIH). It is a seminal report providing state-of-the-art information and perspectives, and it clearly issues a challenge to destigmatize the whole area of mental health and to move on to apply our existing knowledge to "usher in a healthy era of mind and body for the nation." We draw heavily from this report in this chapter, and unashamedly so, because it represents perhaps the best compilation at this time of the established data in the field of mental health.

In the past few decades, mental health research has advanced by leaps and bounds. The basic neurosciences have given us a much more detailed understanding of the complexities inside the brain. Behavioral science has moved beyond description to prescription and new modalities of intervention have been introduced. In addition, pharmaceutical research has brought new drugs with more specificity and fewer side effects, into the market place. Yet we still have a long way to go in understanding the fundamental mechanisms that determine thought, emotion and behavior – and perhaps moreso, a better understanding of what goes wrong in the brain to cause mental illness. After all, the brain is the control center – the integrator, the compiler – of all the functions in the body. It governs thought, emotion, behavior *and health*.

MIND-BODY CONTINUUM

As research has progressed, the detailed information that we have gained about molecular biology in the brain on the one hand, then through the visceral physiology of other body organs and systems, right up to and including emotion, behavior and social interaction on the other – all this has confirmed that any polarized distinction between mind and body is at best formal, and at worst, false. Mental health and physical health are organically connected through brain function.

The false distinction probably dates back to the seventeenth century when the French philosopher Rénè Descartes, conceptualized the distinction between the mind and the body. In his formulation, the so-called 'mind' was completely separable from the 'body' (or 'matter', in general terms). In fact, he thought the mind (and spirit) was the concern and domain of organized religion, whereas the body was the interest of physicians. That term 'mind' itself has been subject to many interpretations over time but a general definition today might be 'the totality of mental functions relating to thinking, mood and purposive behavior.' As such it derives from activities in the brain, but it may indeed have characteristics which emerge beyond the total sum of individual neurological functions. This would include for example, self-consciousness and moral consciousness.

The point goes beyond the philosophy and semantics, to underscore that brain activity does directly impact the health of the body and vice versa. Mental functions are physical and biological; **what happens in the 'mind' directly influences what happens in the body and the same in reverse**. That is the rationale for psychopharmacology, both legal and illegal. It makes sense of something as simple and yet as elusive as the experience of nightmares after going to sleep with a full stomach. Or conversely, waking up in the midst of a nightmare with shortness of breath, a racing heart and sweaty palms. Even in the normal course of daily activity, our attitudes and thought life impact cardiac function, stomach acid secretion, acneform skin lesions etc. Similarly, sufferers of chronic pain are prone to depression and exposure to stress causes anxiety, while toxic chemicals can be triggers of psychosis. The neuroscientist Candice Pert who discovered the opiate receptor, states it clearly, "I can no longer make a clear distinction between the brain and the body." As such, that raises serious questions regarding biological determinism and moral will and responsibility, but such philosophical (or theological) questions are not the purpose here.

What is of importance here is the area of mental health and therefore of mental illness, mental disorder and mental disease. The 'mental' part localizes phenomena in the brain with all its diversity and complexity and 'health' describes a state of successful performance of mental function, resulting in productive activities, fulfilling relationships with other people, and the ability to change and to cope with adversity. 'Illness', 'disorder', and 'disease' are not as easy to distinguish. 'Illness' may be the global term referring to all the diagnosable 'disorders' although these themselves may not include some organic 'diseases' of the brain such as seen in a stroke or in cancer. More importantly though, 'disorders' may be a continuum from the normal activity in the brain leading to normal behavior and cognition – through vague but real and unusual expressions of mood, perception, feeling or behavior that are normal, but yet not pathological – to what becomes then a 'depression', a 'neurosis' a 'psychosis' or 'deviant behavior'. Mental illness is clearly a mix of biological (organic, brain) abnormalities and genetic (or socialized) vulnerabilities to psychosocial stresses. It is a dysfunction of both biochemistry and psychology.

THE BRAIN

The human brain is clearly the most complex structure ever investigated by science. A typical brain weighs only about 3 pounds (or less than 1.5 kilos) and contains billions of conducting nerve cells, or neurons, surrounded by many more supporting cells called glia. These neurons fall into thousands of different types with different chemistry,

shape and connections. Connections are made by tiny, highly specialized structures called synapses. The synapse consists in the first place
of a terminal portion of a 'sending' neuron (the presynapse) which
contains discrete packets of signaling chemicals, or **neurotransmitters**.
Then to communicate, the presynapse, when triggered, releases these
neurotransmitter molecules across the synaptic junction to be received
by the post-synaptic 'receptors' on the so-called dendrites (finger- like
branches) of the second neuron. This is schematically illustrated in
Figure 5. for a particular synapse of relevance to our later discussions
of anxiolytic action.

Figure 5. A Nerve Connection (Synapse)

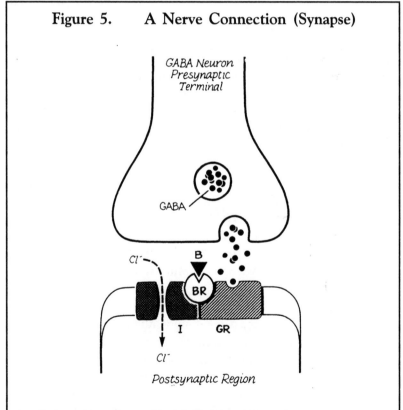

A particular schematic representationof the macromolecular GABAᴀ receptor complex. B = benzodiazepine molecule; I = ionophore containing the
chloride channel; BR = benzodiazepine receptor; GR = GABA receptor.

Structure

The typical neuron has a cell body containing the genetic material and most of its energy producing machinery. From the cell body there is usually a long single branch called the axon, down which signals are transmitted out. The axon may divide near the end into many terminals for connections. Also emanating from the cell body are the branches (or dentrites) which assume very many shapes and sizes, all relevant to the way that incoming messages are processed. It is estimated that each neuron on average, makes over 1000 synaptic connections with other neurons and some as many as 100,000 to 200,000. But each of these trillions of synapses is highly specialized to create in total, an architecture of integrated circuits that makes the best electronic computer today like a mere trivial toy, by comparison. In these circuits, both large and small, electrical charges travel down the axons of pre-synaptic neurons and trigger the chemical release of the neurotransmitters which then diffuse across the synapses, to initiate more electrical signals in the post-synaptic neurons.

These integrated circuits are further organized so that information is processed simultaneously along parallel streams which interpret different types of data. A single visual input from meeting another person, for example, can be processed for shape, size, identity, color, association, value, emotion, ... etc. But none of this is random. The brain is structured for function, such that each locus is specialized for assigned tasks. New imaging technologies such as functional magnetic resonance imaging (MRI) and positron emission tomography (PET) have greatly expanded our knowledge of brain structure and function in recent years.

Grossly, the brain is divided into three main sections, the largest is the cerebrum, then the cerebellum a little lower at the back, and finally the brain stem which connects to the spinal cord. The cerebrum is in two main halves (right and left brain) and on section, has an outer cortex like a mantle of neurons outside the white matter, which in turn surrounds the grey matter. The cortex processes a lot of sensual input and information in different areas, and in the frontal area, the highest integrated brain functions take place. The 'white matter' consists of large numbers of axons covered by the myelin insulator sheaths. The 'grey matter' (like the cortex) contains again many cell bodies. It includes for example, the basal ganghia involved in initiating motion (and therefore the key site in Parkinson's disease) and in integrating motivational states (therefore relevant to addiction). It also includes **the amygdala** (which is involved in anxiety and other emotional states) and **the hippocampus** (with responsibilities such as encoding memory). More particularly for what follows, it also includes the **thalamus** and **hypothalamus**. These are relatively small regions of the total brain but they have many important functions, some of which are central to what we will discuss later. The thalamus is a large ovoid mass of grey matter situated on either side of a fluid chamber called the third ventricle. It has very important sensory and motor functions and acts like a giant relay station. The hypothalamus lies just below the thalamus and it has a very important role in the neuro-endocrine system – that is, the complete communication network of nerves and hormones ... These are just a few chosen examples of the many and varied critical structures in the gray matter of the brain.

To summarize, the brain has a vast number of neurons that communicate continuously and are arranged in parallel integrated circuits that form a structural pattern, such that geographic regions have assigned physiological and psychological functions. There is now, a fairly well understood structure – function relationship. This is anatomy; this is physiology; this is *science*. It is not fancy speculation or romantic notions about *nature*.

Function

In addition to this complexity of architecture, there is a chemical complexity in the brain as highlighted by the more than 100 different neurotransmitter substances. These molecules fall into two major classes: some are small molecules like dopamine, serotonin or norepinephrine (adrenaline); and others are larger peptides (protein chains) like the endogenous opiates (endorphins), substance P (notorious in pain fibres), and corticotropin–releasing hormone (CRH).

The neurotransmitter is released from the pre-synaptic neuron when triggered. It crosses the synapse and attaches to tailor-made protein receptors to initiate a biological effect and subsequent electrical signal. Each neurotransmitter has a number of different kinds of receptors which may trigger different events in the receiving neuron.

Receptors can also be divided into two broad classes. The first class are called ligand-gated receptors because on binding the 'ligand' (neurotransmitter) a pore within *or adjacent to* the receptor molecule itself is opened, and electric charges enter the receiving neuron or cell. That can activate other ion channels that allow more charges to enter. Beyond some threshold, the cell then fires an action potential – an electrical 'discharge' which causes the release of the neurotransmitter. Neurotransmitters that admit positive charges, classically the amino acid 'glutamate', are excitatory. Conversely, other neurotransmitters, on interaction with their receptors, permit negative charges into the cell, thereby reducing its potential and 'inhibiting' firing. The classic neuroinhibitory transmitter is another amino acid called **gamma amino butyric acid (GABA).** The corresponding GABA receptor is the most abundant receptor in the brain. This is a key to what follows later.

The second major class of neurotransmitters interact with receptors which are neither clearly excitatory or inhibiting. Rather, they interact with signaling proteins – called 'G-proteins' – and the receptors are called G-protein-linked-receptors. They then exert important modulating influences on the receiver neuron.

The first class of receptors are found in the circuits that carry specific input data and/or are involved with precise point-to-point communication in the brain such as found in the visual or auditory cortex. These follow a very exact pattern of rapid firing (in milliseconds).

The second major class of much fewer receptors that modulate these precise circuits are apparently confined to a limited number of areas in the brain. It is estimated that only 1 in 200,000 neurons in the brain make dopamine for example, and even fewer make serotonin. But their effects are critical. Although their cell bodies are clustered, they have axons with branches that traverse the entire brain so that their modulating influences are felt everywhere. They are therefore critical targets for chemical interventions such as anxiolytic, antidepressant or antipsychotic drugs – as well as active sites for illegal drug abuse.

Although structure and function are so intimately correlated in the brain, the situation is always changing. Daily experiences cause new neurons to develop and new synaptic connections to be made, as in evolving software. Life demands the ability to grow, to recall and to cope with an ever-changing environment, and the brain rises to the challenge. The net result is more than the sum expression of the 50,000 plus genes that design and build it. It is also the product of one's environment from early gestation and beyond. Hence, there is hope for healing and health even when mental illness is apparent, through wise and targeted interventions. The biological description of the brain is not necessarily 'deterministic' and it can guide us to develop treatments for mental illness that are more effective and with fewer side effects.

MENTAL ILLNESS CHARACTERISTICS

Mental status forms yet another true continuum – one between what is totally normal and healthy, and that which is diagnosable as disorder. To clarify the situation, a systematic approach to the classification and diagnosis of mental illness has been developed (The U.S. manual *Diagnostic and Statistical Manual of Mental Disorders* is in its fourth edition –DSM-IV (1994) from the American Psychiatric Association).

Mental health was traditionally neglected by doctors as late as the early to mid-twentieth century. But with the discovery of psychoactive drugs that clearly indicated that mental illness was an illness in the truest sense, it has gained more attention in the mainstream of healthcare. Developments in both neuroscience and behavioral science have led to major advances in the past fifty years so that the reliable diagnosis, effective treatment, quality of life and prognosis of those who suffer from mental illness have all dramatically improved. Yet the public at large has still been slow to eliminate the associated stigma and to afford the mentally ill the respect and dignity they deserve. More and more, these patients are able to conduct very normal lives.

Yet the prevalence of mental illness is always underestimated, since many who suffer from its effect never seek help, never get diagnosed, never get treated. Yet it is estimated that one in every four or five persons in North America is vulnerable to a diagnosable mental disorder each year. Mental disorders collectively account for more than 15 percent of the overall burden of disease from *all* causes, ranking second, and with a slightly higher burden than that associated with all forms of cancer. Major depression is the leading cause of disability in the United States and in the extreme form, suicide is the seventh leading cause of death.

For simplicity we have summarized the major areas of mental illness in Table 6. Categories are defined by the major class of signs or symptoms manifested in each case, although these tend to overlap quite often. We shall discuss these major symptoms of mental disorders in turn and then go on to treatment methods.

Anxiety

Anxiety is a very common symptom. It is a normal reaction to the stressors of everyday life. It can be a simple nervous response to speaking in public, writing an exam or doing an interview. Or it could be a sudden intense fear in response to some threatening experience like just missing an accident, or a positive diagnostic test, or a strange policeman's knock at the door. Such experiences provoke reactions like a feeling of fear or dread, rapid heart rate, trembling, restlessness and muscle tension, light headedness, cold hands/feet, irritability, stomach upset, and/or shortness of breath. But the experience is precipitous, short-lived and easily reversible. It is probably a survival mechanism, alerting mind and body of immediate threats to safety or survival. It is part of the general adaptation syndrome in response to stress – a preparation for fight or flight. It arouses you to action and helps you cope.

But **anxiety** can be a mental disorder when this reaction is exaggerated or inordinate, it is no longer positive and helpful, it can be just the opposite. It can keep a person from coping and disrupt one's daily life. It then becomes more than a case of 'nerves.' It becomes an illness, related to one's biological makeup (in the brain) and their life experiences. When persistent and unrealistic worry becomes a habitual style of life, a way of approaching situations, an individual may be suffering from *generalized anxiety disorder (GAD)*.

Anxiety is aroused most intensely by some immediate physical threat to one's safety, but it also occurs commonly in response to dangers that are relatively remote or abstract. Even intense anxiety can result from situations that one can only vaguely imagine or anticipate. The key element of GAD is the persistent worry that is unrelated to any other illness and disproportionate to any real threat. It is more than 'butterflies in the stomach' since it is a real, medical illness that can have real physical symptoms and destroy one's quality of life. Any

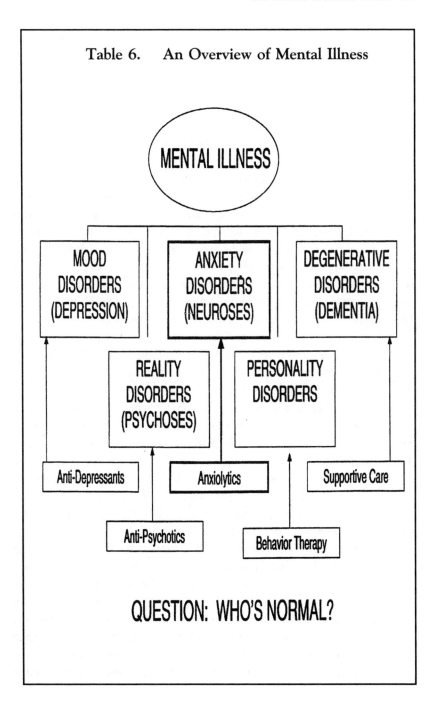

Table 6.   An Overview of Mental Illness

QUESTION: WHO'S NORMAL?

chronic and excessive worry about events that are unlikely to occur is cause for concern. The formal DSM-IV Diagnostic Criteria for GAD is shown in Table 7. Other generalized anxiety is a more diffuse and non-specific kind of anxiety experienced as excessive worrying, restlessness, and tension occurring with a chronic and sustained pattern. Other inappropriate expressions of anxiety include phobias, panic attacks, obsessive-compulsive disorder (OCD), and post traumatic stress disorder (PTSD).

Individuals with **phobias** experience high-level anxiety when exposed to specific situations or objects that can vary widely. Social phobias usually arise in childhood or adolescence and can be chronic and disabling. Simple phobias produce an immediate anxiety response on exposure to the stimulus and the anticipatory anxiety leads to phobic avoidance of the object or situation.

Panic attacks are brief but very intense bouts of anxiety, triggered by almost any kind of stimulus, whether sensual or imagined. These could be as common as perfumes or hair sprays or be more specialized such as the high levels of carbon monoxide found in crowded airplanes or elevators. During the attack there are multiple symptoms indicative of uncontrolled physiological changes (autonomic dysfunction) and usually a feeling of impending doom, or a fear that one is having a heart attack or some other serious illness. This type usually begins in early adult life and tends to be chronic in nature, with exacerbations and remissions. Some 5-10 percent of the population are affected at some time in life.

Obsessive-compulsive disorder (OCD) individuals have fixed action patterns that they repeat anxiously with little real justification e.g. hand-washing, checking the stove. etc. Their high level of anxiety drives them to obsessional thinking or to compulsive behavior. There is a realization on the patient's part that the action is unreasonable and a product of their own mind, but they are unable to resist performing the action without marked anxiety. It is frequently associated with depression and has its onset in adolescence or early adult life.

Post-traumatic stress disorder (PTSD) is a product of some intense and overwhelming fearful event that leads to repetitious and persistent re-experiencing of the same in memories and dreams. It also produces deliberate avoidance of associated stimuli and increased arousal.

Table 7. Diagnostic Criteria (DSM-IV) for Generalized Anxiety Disorder (GAD)

A. Unrealistic or excessive anxiety and worry about life circumstances for a period greater than 6 months, during which this person has been bothered by theses concerns for more days than not.

B. The person has difficulty controlling the anxiety and worrying

C. The anxiety and worry are associated with at least 3 of the following symptoms:
   1. Restlessness or feeling keyed up or on edge
   2. Being easily fatigued
   3. Difficulty concentrating or mind going blank
   4. Irritability
   5. Muscle tension
   6. Sleep disturbances

D. If another psychiatric disorder is present, the focus of the anxiety and worry is unrelated to it.

E. The anxiety, worry, or physical symptoms cause significant distress or impairment in social, occupational, or some other important aspect of functioning.

F. The disturbance is not due to the direct effect of a substance, medication, or general medical condition, and does not occur only during the course of a mood disorder, a psychotic disorder, or a pervasive development disorder.

Not everyone develops PTSD after exposure to such a traumatic or fearful event. On average, about 9 percent do, but estimates are higher for particular types of trauma such as female victims of crime.

Whatever the manifestation of anxiety, there is an apparent loss of control or regulation of the otherwise normal stress reaction. This has an organic basis in brain function and responds to pharmacotherapy as well as to behavioral therapy and cognitive-behavioral therapy.

More than 19 million Americans suffer from an anxiety

disorder each year, making this category **the most prevalent of all mental illnesses**. The lifetime risk for an anxiety disorder is nearly 25 percent. But it is estimated that less than one third of sufferers receive appropriate treatment. Much too often, anxiety disorders have been trivialized and moreover, sufferers have been stigmatized and labeled as the 'worried well'. But anxiety disorders are real mental illnesses that exact a tremendous toll both on individuals and society as a whole. Although estimates of the associated healthcare costs reach $42 billion a year in the United States (similar to the estimated annual costs for clinical depression) much of this has been shown to be attributable to misdiagnosis and undertreatment. More than half that cost derives from repeated inappropriate use of healthcare services, since these patients are 3-5 times more likely to visit their doctor and 6 times more likely to be hospitalized. In addition, about 43 percent of people with anxiety disorder are also depressed or abuse alcohol or drugs. Use of psychiatric services account for 31 per cent of the total annual cost, and loss of productivity at work, including absenteeism, accounts for another 10 percent. Early diagnosis of underlying anxiety disorders and appropriate management could reduce healthcare costs and increase productivity in the workplace.

Mood

Mood is a relatively simple, intuitive concept but a difficult entity to formulate in scientific terms. It is essentially a subjective quality – an internal feeling that gets expressed in an **affect** which can in turn be observed. Moods vary in each individual over time and everyone understands what it is to feel sad at some times and to be happy at other times. Particular neurotransmitters in the brain, and some parts of the brain more than others, do have a direct impact on the experience of mood, which is generally modulated or regulated in a healthy individual to avoid sustained feelings at either extreme.

Disturbances of mood characteristically manifest themselves as sustained feelings of sadness or sustained elevation of mood. In either case there is a dysregulation of mood – a failure to control the exaggerated feeling. It is a sense of being carried along by an internal wave of emotion either downward into sadness, hopelessness and even despair, or upward in exhilaration and overdrive. The operative phrase of that metaphor is being *carried along* by the turbulence with little sense of control and the inability to modulate the amplitude. It is not some inherent personal weakness that one can change at will by "pulling yourself together". It is an illness with biological components, if not actual causes.

These disturbances of mood can occur in different patterns associated with different mental disorders. The most common of these is associated with persistent sadness and constitutes a **major depression**. That associated with the sustained elevation or extreme fluctuation of mood is **bipolar disorder**. Less extreme versions of these disorders are called **dysthymia** and **hypomania** respectively.

Each of these mood disorders have characteristic symptoms and signs commonly associated with them. They may be grouped for convenience to form an acronym in each case (Table 8).

Table 8.	Common Symptoms Associated With Mood Disorders
Depression	**Bipolar Disorder**
Sleep disturbance, up or down	Ideas in flight, thoughts racing
Interest decline, in pleasure and sex	Grandiose thinking, egotism
Guilt feelings, unwarranted	Over involvement, sex
Mood: sad all or most of the time	Talkative, pressured speech
Energy levels low	Sleep decline
Cognitive impairment, concentration low	Activity increased, restlessness
Psychomotor retardation	Distractibility
Suicidal ideation	

Along with the pervasive feelings of sadness or elatedness, these mood disorders are commonly associated with a variety of symptoms that relate to vegetative functions (appetite, sleep, sex, energy) and to cognitive functions (concentration, memory, judgement) as well as behavioral patterns (withdrawal, anti-social) and more. Why such a diversity of symptoms is not yet clear, but it is tempting to suggest that common neurotransmitters and/or receptors may be involved or some common secondary modulatory circuits as we described earlier. In healthy individuals (or higher organisms for that matter) the complex group of responses and behaviors that constitute mood must be subject to precise and tightly controlled regulation. That allows for adaptation to the many changing environments and demands at any given time. A depressed mood might then reflect a type of global damping (modulation) of these vegetative and cognitive functions, while a manic state may reflect the excessive activation of these same functions.

In any case, there are well established DSM-IV criteria for clear diagnosis of affective (mood) disorders. These criteria do not assume any specific etiology (or cause) for the disorder. They require no model per se. In fact, while a major depression may be triggered by some particular life circumstance or event, the mood reaction seems greatly exaggerated. In all likelihood, depression has less to do with events that occur than with an individual's inherent vulnerability to the condition. The precipitating factor(s) combine with the pre-disposing factor(s) to cause the depressive episode. Unfortunately, although up to 18-20 million North Americans suffer from some type of depression, many of these (nearly two-thirds) do not recognize their illnesses, do not seek help or find effective relief. In terms of human suffering, the consequences of untreated depression are beyond measure. They include loss of self-esteem, abuse of alcohol and drugs, family and career disruption, chronic disability and in many cases, death (particularly in the young and the elderly). The good news is that more than 80 percent of people suffering from mood disorders (depression) can be successfully treated.

Psychosis

Psychosis is a broad category of symptoms resulting from disturbances of perception and thought. The psychotic person has a **grossly impaired sense of reality**, often coupled with emotional and cognitive disabilities, which severely compromises their ability to function. Clearly, psychosis is a matter of degree and the threshold will vary to some degree in different cultural settings. It is not a single disorder but a group of syndromes depending on the groupings of the various symptoms.

Generally, the individual with a psychotic disorder will tend to talk and act in strange or bizarre fashion. **Schizophrenia** is the typical example. It has little to do with dual personality as so many believe, but essentially with the loss of reality. It tends to have familial pattern suggesting a genetic component. The symptoms often appear at a younger age and to recur from time to time even with treatment. It can and often does lead to a marked deterioration in social and occupational functioning. The condition affects one in every 1000-2000 people and the lifetime risk is as high as one percent. It tends to be more common in lower socioeconomic classes but this may reflect the consequences as much as the cause. Brief reactive psychoses could be episodes of less than two weeks duration; schizophrenia disorders are described up to six months and for classic schizophrenia, the duration must be at least six months and not associated with any specific organic disease.

In the normal individual, sensory information is processed and interpreted in the brain in a coherent and realistic fashion. When those brain activities fail to function properly, one can experience a wide range of unusual perceptions and thoughts that depart from reality. A common group of such symptoms are the **hallucinations.** These occur when a person experiences sensory impressions that are quite real to them but are totally subjective. They could involve any sensory modality such as hearing voices, seeing things, smelling aromas, touching or being touched and even tasting flavors or foods. Note, these are sensory in nature. **Delusions**, on the other hand, are false beliefs or constructs that a person might hold despite all evidence to the contrary. There is now a disordered interpretation of information, a failure in thought processing. **Paranoia** is a common example, where an individual is convinced that others are trying to harm them. They cannot be convinced otherwise for their conclusion (delusion) is not related to the facts of any situation.

In addition to hallucinations and delusions, victims of psychotic disorder may have thought processes that are characteristically loose, disorganized, illogical or bizarre. Naturally, such disturbances in thought often lead to similar disorganized and bizarre patterns of behavior. These symptoms all reflect malfunction in the content and process of thinking and as such are *positive symptoms*.

Another group of symptoms seen in patients with psychoses reflect major deficits in motivation and spontaneity. Something is lacking here. It is the absence of thoughts and behaviors that one could normally expect and so this group is referred to as *negative symptoms*. They include a flat or blunted affect, poverty of speech, the inability to experience any normal pleasure (anhedonia), poor motivation, lack of spontaneity or initiative. There is also the tendency to think only in concrete terms because the ability to think abstractly, outside the sensory world, is grossly impaired.

In general terms, it is noteworthy that the positive symptoms like hallucinations or delusions, are responsible for much of the acute distress associated with schizophrenia, whereas the negative symptoms like loss of motivation or initiative, can be responsible for so much of the chronic and long term disability associated with these disorders.

The psychotic symptoms derive from the failure in the brain and central nervous system to process and interpret information. They obviously have common mechanisms of pathopysiology and it is not surprising that they tend to respond as a group to the specific pharmacological interventions which are used to manage these patients. What is surprising is the acute response observed when a psychotic person who may present in the emergency room as loud, boisterous, agitated, acting bizarre and almost uncontrollable – when given a neuroleptic drug, within minutes can be as different as night and day – subdued, quiet, cooperative, peaceful but still detached. This single scientific intervention has transformed mental health facilities.

Cognition

One of the most sophisticated activities of the brain is the general ability to organize, process, store and retrieve information. We are capable of acquiring knowledge, retaining it, and retrieving it on demand. Think of perceiving, recognizing, conceiving, judging, sensing, reasoning and imagining. The sum total we call *cognition*. Each of the cognitive tasks relates to specific functions in the brain which are activated depending on the nature of information conceived, perceived or retrieved, and the circumstances surrounding it at the time. Furthermore, there are many associated functions such as the ability to execute a complex sequence of tasks. We not only know *what,* but we know *why* and we know *how*, and we integrate it all.

Disturbances of cognitive function can occur in a variety of disorders. The most pertinent today in our aging society is the progressive deterioration that we call **dementia.** This may be caused by several specific conditions including Alzheimer's disease, mini-strokes, alcoholism, infection, vitamin deficiency, chemical poisoning (as in severe forms of drug addiction), post-traumatic illness, extreme epilepsy, dialysis and more. The most common is Alzheimer's disease (sometimes called senile dementia) which is an organic brain disease characterized clinically by global, progressive and irreversible deterioration of mental or intellectual functioning. This is seen in loss of recent memory (remote memory becomes more difficult in later stages), lability of affect, difficulty with novel experience, self-centeredness and repeated childish behavior. Just as in children - attention, concentration and higher intellectual functions are significantly impaired. Also, language difficulties range from the difficulty in finding a particular word to the complete inability to speak coherently or to understand what is being heard. Even the simplest activities of daily living like bathing and dressing become difficult to impossible, making demands on caregivers and support services.

Impairment of cognitive function can often occur in other mental conditions, particularly depression, and increasingly so with age. It is sometimes quite difficult to distinguish this 'pseudodementia' as a sign of depression from the real degenerative condition that is true Alzheimer's. But a careful mental status examination, with particular attention to the 'quality' of responses can afford a proper diagnosis. In any case, pathological findings of cerebral atrophy (the brain shrinks), increased senile plaques, neurofibrillary tangles and granulovacuolar degeneration are characteristic signs of Alzheimer's. Biochemically, there are multiple changes, with a consistent deficiency of choline acetyl transferase, a key enzyme for the neurotransmitter acetyl choline. Other neurotransmitters are clearly affected.

The prevalence of Alzheimer's disease in the elderly, the aging of the population and the demands on the healthcare system that these patients make (whether at home or in institutions), demand that efforts to further understand and manage this illness become a high priority as we begin this new century.

Other Symptoms

We have outlined the most important manifestations of mental illness: anxiety, mood disturbances, psychosis and cognitive degenerative disorders. But that leaves large areas of human behavior and experience out of the picture. We have not addressed issues of relevance to children like autism, speech and language disorders, learning disability, sleep disorders, attention deficit disorders, and stereotyped movement disorders. Neither have we looked at the wide area of personality disorders which include all those enduring maladaptive patterns of behavior that cause difficulty with relationships in all aspects of living – in the family, at work, in recreation and even with oneself. Similarly, we have omitted disorders as basic and as common as the serious eating disorders, the sexual and gender identity disorders, and disorders related to impulse-control. All these and more are beyond the scope of this chapter and indeed, of this book.

The primary focus here is to demonstrate the basic scientific background underlying our contemporary knowledge of mental health so that we do not fall into the trap of waving our hands, dreaming of *natural* solutions and making false and exaggerated claims with respect to novel interventions for mental health, which is clearly so important to any consideration of Wellness.

We will now turn our attention then, more specifically to what we know about the cause or etiology of these disorders in general, then in the next Chapter we will consider the anxiety disorders in particular. We will then go on to address the question of treatment and how anxiolytic drugs work. This will form the basis for the novel research report regarding the technological breakthrough of harvesting another miracle ingredient from nature's goldmine, which is the subject of the following chapter.

ORIGINS OF MENTAL ILLNESS

The fact that mental health and mental illness are directly determined by brain function should not imply that only the biological factors are important. Clearly human behavior and experience involve the important psychological, social and cultural influences on each individual. The psychological and sociocultural phenomena are indeed represented in the brain, through memories and learning. These involve structural changes in the brain cell neurons and the neuronal circuits.

Much of what we know about the origins of mental disorders is derived from noticing correlations or associations between any given disorder and one or more events or incidences. This correlation usually assesses risk, which allows us to identify 'risk factors'. To determine causation, the hallmark is the randomized, double-blind controlled experiment (RCT) such as we described in Chapter Three. But particularly in mental health, such experimental research on humans is often very difficult, if not impossible, because of logistics, ethics or cost. A reasonable biological understanding can often be gained from animal studies if appropriate models can be found to simulate what may often be real behavior patterns and functioning, otherwise attributable to humans themselves. Such models do indeed exist.

The correlations and causes for any disorder must be further distinguished from the consequences observed as later outcomes of that disorder. For example, the fact that schizophrenia is more common among the lower socioeconomic class is a well-recognized *correlation*. Is there something amongst that class of people that causes schizophrenia? One might think of diet, accessibility and use of healthcare, environmental exposure at home or at work, and so on, as possible contributing *causes*. But on the other hand, there is a tendency for schizophrenic patients to be ostracized, discriminated against with respect to employment, housing and so on, which causes them to drift downward in society and their prevalence in the lower socioeconomic class maybe nothing more than a *consequence* of their illness. So then the real question arises: is the linkage between schizophrenia and lower socioeconomic class a mere correlation only, a true cause, or a real consequence? That's the complexity of the association.

But in biological terms, there are known biological and physical factors that contribute to mental health and disease. These include genes, infections, physical trauma, nutrition, hormones and certainly, toxins. The genetic influence is very important because the degree of sophistication and complexity of brain functioning would clearly amplify the minutest of changes at the molecular level. But the majority of mental disorders arise in part from defects of multiple genes and not any single one. These multiple genes increase only the risk of mental illness.

The inherent risk is converted into an observed disorder when those genes interact with environmental factors, including both physical exposure and experience.

The psychosocial factors that influence mental health and disease are quite diverse. The psychological ones must include all the stressful life events, the baseline affect which reflects one's mood and level of arousal, personality, and of course gender. The social influences involve parents, the racial, cultural and religious background, socioeconomic status, interpersonal relationships and their course, and much, much more. To get a grip on all these diverse psychosocial influences, theories have been developed including the psychodynamic theories of personality, best known by Freudian psychoanalysis; and theories of behaviorism and social learning which gave rise to the more recent cognitive-behavioral therapy.

So much for mental-illness, in general. What we intend to explore as we go searching in nature's goldmine for another important nugget, is in the area of anxiety and coping with the stressors of life. After all, we pointed out earlier that this is the most prevalent form of mental illness and grossly undertreated, at least in any formal or effective terms. But as we shall see, the alternative health care practitioners recognize the importance of this to the 'whole person' and often advocate solutions from *nature* that do no justice to the science we already know regarding mental health. And there is a better way which we shall soon discover.

Now we can turn to anxiety disorders in particular.

Chapter Eight

ANXIETY: IT'S CAUSE & CURE

Mechanisms

From the foregoing observations on mental illness, you would expect anxiety to be the product of biological, psychological and social factors. And that it certainly is. Anxiety disorders are heterogeneous and still not fully understood but we do know that some, like panic disorder, have a stronger biological (presumably genetic) cause, while others derive more from life experiences. We do know that women have higher rates of most anxiety disorders than men do, but that is still a correlation, not necessarily a contributing cause.

Several different theories have been advanced to attempt an explanation of what causes anxiety. Most of these are essentially psychosocial in perspective with little or no appreciation for the likely organic roots of the phenomenon.

The psychosocial views of anxiety disorders focus on different aspects of individual *conflicts* and conditioning. The psychodynamic theories perceive the associated symptoms as an expression of underlying conflicts. Anxiety is seen to reflect basic, unresolved conflicts in one's value system, or in intimate relationships or in expression of anger. Behavioral theories see unpredictable positive and negative *reinforcement* (think of Pavlor's dogs) leading to anxiety when one is unsure about whether avoidance behaviors are effective. Cognitive factors also play a critical role, especially the way in which people interpret or think about stressful events. One is overwhelmed by apparent *loss of control*. They become helpless when they cannot predict, control or guarantee their desired results. This type of vulnerability becomes then pathological.

The ubiquitous characteristic of anxiety disorders is the state of increased arousal or fear. It is the extreme, exaggerated, overblown 'fight or flight' response that we referred to earlier. That normal acute stress response has been well studied in animals. It shows characteristic physiological changes consistent with the activation of a particular nucleus in the brain called the **locus ceruleus**. This was the presumed **anatomical basis**. The tiny shallow depression lies at the base of the brain near the so-called cerebral aqueduct, and contains about 20,000 melanin-pigmented neuronal cell bodies. It is the origin of most norepinephrine (noradrenulin) pathways in the brain. The neurons that use this neurotransmitter leave that nucleus and extend along distinct pathways to the cerebral cortex, the limbic system, the cerebellum, and down the spinal cord, among others. In a tranquil state, these neurons "fire" minimally. In the *first pathway* of activation, sensory input to the sensory cortex of the brain is relayed through the thalamus to the brain stem, increasing the rate of 'firing' in the locus ceruleus en route. This makes the animal alert and attentive to the environment. When a threat is perceived, the discharge becomes intense and prolonged and the norepinephrine drives the autonomic nervous system into high gear: the heart, blood vessels, respiratory centers etc. The *second pathway* involved is via the hypothalamus which secretes hormones to the pituitary gland, which secretes other hormones to the adrenal gland, which then pours out more noreprinephrine (noradrenalin). This combination of neuronal and hormonal activation guarantees an adequate acute stress response to defend life and limb when threatened.

Up to the 1980's, most scientists believed that anxiety was due mainly to the excess discharge of the locus ceruleus in the acute stress response. But it is now clear that the acute stress response is really an *arousal*, and arousal and anxiety are not the same thing. Furthermore, anxiolytic drugs tend to act on different neurotransmitters and receptor sites – namely GABA and serotonin, not norepinephrine (noradrenalin) or epinephrine (adrenalin). Research has now shown that the locus ceruleus still participates in anxiety, but to a much lesser extent than was believed for a long time.

More recent research has pointed in a different direction. The focus of anxiety biology is now on two key regulatory centers found in the cerebral hemispheres of the brain – the **hippocampus** and the

amygdala. They regulate the second or hypothalamic – pituatary – adrenocortical (HPA) axis referred to above. They are major nuclei of the so-called **limbic system** which describes a heterogeneous array of brain structures at or near the edge (or limbus) of the medial wall of the cerebral hemisphere. The term is also used to denote the visceral brain (i.e. the part controlling body organs). More particularly here, it sometimes also includes the interconnections between these nuclei as well as their connections with the septal area, the hypothalamus and other areas. These latter connections become a pathway for regulatory influence and control of the endocrine (hormonal) and autonomic nervous and motor systems, as well as a factor in motivational and mood states.

The hippocampus (derived from the Greek term for a 'sea horse' because of its shape) is a structure producing a prominent elevation on the floor of the inferior horn of the lateral ventricle at the base of the brain. It is considered important in verbal memory, especially of time and place for events with strong emotional overtones.

The amygdala (derived again from the Greek term for 'almond' or Latin for 'tonsil') has been identified with fear responses. There is good evidence for this from non-invasive neuroimaging. Sensory input is to the lateral side where it is processed and passed to the central nucleus which produces the major output from the amygdala. The neurons that leave there project to multiple brain systems which are involved with the physiological and behavioral responses to fear. In particular, the projections to different regions in the hypothalamus activate the sympathetic nervous system and induce the release of stress hormones, including corticotropin-releasing hormone (CRH). The release of CRH in turn triggers a cascade leading to the release of the glucocorticoids from the adrenal cortex. Other projections affect pain response (increasing tolerance to the point that anxious people such as wounded soldiers or athletes can do the unthinkable) or other defensive responses specific to different animals (e.g. some freeze by reflex when afraid). Further research on these pathways is on-going.

We commented above that **anxiety is different from fear**. Anxiety is in the anticipation of some danger or threat which causes the same arousal, vigilance, 'fight or flight' physiology, and associated negative effects and cognition. Research continues to elucidate if and how the dysregulation of these normal fear pathways gives rise to the observed anxiety disorders. Neuroimaging has already afforded direct evidence in humans of the damaging effects of glucocorticoids. Such studies have shown that there is a definite reduction in size of the hippocampus in victims of post-traumatic stress disorder (PTSD) referred to earlier. Further, this reduced volume may reflect the atrophy or wasting of the dendrites – recall the receptive portion of nerve cells – in a select region of the hippocampus. Likewise, animals that were exposed to chronic psychosocial stress, show similar wasting in the same region of their hippocampus. This atrophy is presumed to be associated with the stress-induced glucocorticoids. The implication would then be that if the hippocampus is impaired, the person would be less able to draw on their memory to evaluate the exact nature of the external or internal stressor. Such would be an anatomical basis for anxiety.

The more **biochemical basis** for anxiety disorders would go to the level of neurotransmitters, of which at least five are known to be involved: serotonin, norepinephrine, gamma-aminobutyric acid (GABA), corticotropin-releasing hormone (CRH) and now cholecystokinin. These obviously interact by what are called feedback mechanisms. Of special interest here, we emphasize that GABA and serotonin are known **inhibitory** neurotransmitters that quiet the stress response. Note too, that GABA is by far the most abundant inhibitory neurotransmitter in the brain, estimated to act at 25% of all the synapses in the neocortex and cerebellum. These are therefore obvious targets for anxiolytic drugs which now leads us to a further understanding of this inhibitory mechanism.

ANXIOLYTIC DRUGS

Mental disorders are treatable. In fact, for most mental disorders there is generally a number of different treatments which have been proven effective. Some estimates put the overall success rate as high as 80 percent for those who come into treatment, especially with using both drugs and different kinds of psychosocial therapy. But sadly, less than one-third of adults with a diagnosable mental disorder, and it is even less for children, receive any mental health services in a given year. There is now an all-out effort to bring more of these victims into the mental healthcare system which can deliver so much healing and help.

The Tranquilization of America

In contrast to the denial and negligence just referred to, several generations of Americans since the last World War have turned to drugs – legal and illegal – with the expectations that new pills would make them happy, restful, less depressed, better workers and yes, better lovers.

Wallace Laboratories and Wyeth laboratories began marketing an anti-anxiety drug known generically as meprobamate and in the consumer market as **Miltown**™ and Equanil™. In those days, Miltown was credited with reducing anxiety and stress, without side effects. However, it later proved to be addictive and to show dangerous interactions with other drugs. In any case, it was a major advance over earlier sedatives and narcotics which had major potential side effects. It only took months to invade the American popular culture especially after the TV comedian *Milton* Berle made fun of himself as '*Miltown* Berle'. It was popularized in bestselling magazines and within one year, 5 percent of the American population was taking tranquilizers.

Ensuing competition gave rise to the Benzheptoxdiazines, a different class of drugs from a different company – the Swiss based pharmaceutical group, Hoffman-LaRoche. These were substances originally used in the dyeing industry, but by 1960, chlordiazepoxide or **Librium**™ hit the market. The name said it all, a short form for "equilibrium". Soon, the Hoffman-LaRoche chemists would come with the new and improved sequel which was the first really big benzodiazepine called **Valium**™ (diazepam, 1963). It was stronger and required smaller doses than Librium. Up to 1980, it was the largest-selling pharmaceutical drug in history. By the mid-70's, more than 60 million prescriptions for Valium were being written each year. In 1978, an estimated 20 percent of all women and 14 percent of all men in America were taking Valium. Its popularity was a result of a combination of its pharmacological action, its relative safety and the increased demand for agents of this type by both physicians and patients. But it too proved to be addictive. Its consumption only declined after several media celebrities had their personal struggles publicized before the watching world, and by the start of the 1980's it lost its first-place ranking to an anti-ulcer medication, as the most widely prescribed drug in America.

At the same time, came another big player on the market. It

came as a wide-ranging antidepressant, belonging to a new class of drugs called SSRI's – selective serotonin reuptake inhibitors. This was **Prozac**™ (fluoxetine) which took the market by storm. In its first week, 436,000 prescriptions were reportedly filled. It was designed to keep serotonin in the synapses of brain neurons linked to mood, by preventing the reuptake mechanism. The promoters highlighted its superior safety and widespread efficacy and consumers bought. They got somewhat more than they paid for, because serotonin as we mentioned above is a critical inhibitory neurotransmitter that also impacts the brain circuitry linked to anxiety. So the anti-depressant Prozac also became the anxiolytic Prozac but as we shall show later, the SSRI's prove more effective against particular anxiety disorders whereas benzodiazepines are more suited for patients with Generalized Anxiety Disorder.

Benzodiazepines (Valium™)

Benzodiazepines like Valium are indicated for the management of anxiety disorders or for the short-term relief of the symptoms of anxiety. The anxiety of tension associated with the stress of everyday life usually does not require this type of treatment. Valium is also used in acute alcohol withdrawal to relieve any acute agitation, tremor, impending or acute delirium tremens and hallucinosis. It is also used intravenously in an acute setting to relieve seizures, as well as an adjunct for the relief of skeletal muscle spasm due to reflex spasm to local pathology, such as muscle or joint inflammation, or secondary to trauma.

Valium is contraindicated in patients with known hypersensitivity to the drug and because of insufficient clinical data, in children under 5 or 6 years of age. It is also contraindicated in patients with acute narrow angle glaucoma (usually in the emergency room). It crosses the placenta and should be avoided in pregnancy, especially since congenital malformations have been associated with the use of minor tranquilizers. It should also not be used in conjunction with alcohol and any other CNS-depressant drugs. Finally, it is prudent to avoid any demanding hazardous activity such as operating heavy equipment or extensive driving.

In animals, benzodiazepines were shown to act on the limbic system, the thalamus and hypothalamus, to induce calming effects. These are central effects with no demonstrable autonomic blocking action, and they do not produce what neurologists call 'extra pyramidal' effects. They are relatively safe medications and have rapid and profound effects on anxiety, sedation and sleep. These therapeutic effects are all due to the enhancement of the inhibitory neurotransmitters that use GABA. The benzodiazepines bind to the GABA receptor and increase the inhibitive effect of these neuronal circuits.

The GABA Receptor

At least 90 percent of the GABA in the body is in the central nervous system. GABA itself, its synthetic enzyme and its receptors have been found in all brain regions examined.

GABA is synthesized from the excitatory amino acid, L-glutamic acid, by the specific enzyme L-glutamic acid decarboxylase (GAD), with pyridoxal phosphate (from B6, pyridoxine) as a cofactor. It is removed from the synapse principally by a specific re-uptake mechanism into both nerve terminals and glia cells. It is also metabolized mainly in the glia to form succinate and complete what is called the "GABA shunt".

There are at least two known GABA receptors denoted as $GABA_A$ and $GABA_B$. $GABA_A$ is a macromolecular receptor complex and one of the best studied neurotransmitter synapse mechanisms. It is generally linked to a chloride ion channel and to several other adjacent receptor sites, one of which is the locus for binding the benzodiazepines. The proposed principal mechanism is as follows:

After GABA is synthesized and liberated into the synapse, it interacts with the $GABA_A$ receptor, which causes a specific chloride ion (Cl^-) channel to open. If the receptor is located on a cell body, the channel opening results in hyperpolarization due to increased Cl^- entry; whereas if the contact is axo-axonal (along the nerve fibers), then Cl^- exits from the channel and the result is a local depolarization. Adjacent to the GABA receptor, or at least functionally linked to it, are these other receptor sites including a site for benzodiazepines and a different one for barbiturates. The relative density of these benzodiazepine binding sites in different regions of the human brain, especially the regions of interest to us here, are shown in Table 9. The entire complex (sometimes called **the GABA-chloride ionophore receptor complex**) is involved in the modulation of inhibitory nerve transmission. It has been shown that interaction of benzodiazepines with their specific sites increase chloride conductance in the presence of GABA. What this means is that the benzodiazepines increase or potentiate the inhibitory action of GABA across the synapse.

Table 9.	Relative Density of Benzodiazepine Binding Sites in Different Regions of the Human Brain.	
Region	**Relative Numbers** (per mg protein)	
Cerebral cortex	1200	
Cerebellar cortex	730	
Amygdala	720	
Hippocampus	610	
Hypothalamus	520	

Principles of Medical Pharmacology, fourth edition. Edited by H.Kalant et al., University of Toronto Press (1985)

(Barbiturates have a similar mechanism of action but different chemical effects. There are few recommended uses for barbiturates today even though they were once popular for seizures, insomnia, anesthesia induction and of course, as street drugs. They are no longer considered appropriate for the treatment of either anxiety or insomnia).

It is not clear why these binding sites exist functionally adjacent to the GABAA receptors. Obviously they were not designed for synthetic drugs but rather vice versa. We do know that none of the common neurotransmitters compete for binding there with benzodiazepines. There is no direct effect on the benzodiazepine receptor from norepinephrine (noradrenalin), dopamine, GABA itself, glutamate, glycine or histamine. One suggestion identifies a purine (a nucleic acid base) as a possible endogenous neurotransmitter. There is something else in nature (from nature's goldmine) that will do the trick, but that is the secret of the next chapter.

As so often happens in the world of alternative practitioners, there is a 'rush to judgement' and a simplistic solution to complex problems. Recall from Chapter Six how a market was created for glutathione supplements, once the value of this naturally occurring tripeptide became obvious. But oral glutathione proved ineffective in modulating the intracellular levels of GSH. It was digestible in the gut for one thing and neither GSH itself nor the cysteine precursor were efficient at crossing the cell membrane *into* the cell where its effect was most important. Now, believe it or not, have come ... the GABA promoters. Capsules of GABA are already on the market, being promoted as 'useful in producing a state of relaxation'. They even promote the use of vitamin B-6 with it, because 'GABA works in partnership with a derivative of B-6 (pyridoxine)', to cross from the axons to the dendrites through the synaptic cleft, in response to an electrical signal in the neuron and thereby inhibits message transmission. According to these promoters, this helps control the nerve cells from firing too fast, which would overload the system. Therefore, they reason GABA itself can be taken to calm the body, instead of a tranquilizer and without the fear of addiction. Taken with the B-vitamins niacinamide and inositol, they believe it prevents anxiety messages from reaching the motor centers of the brain by filling its receptor site. That may seem plausible, but it raises a number of important questions which must be answered *before* such clinical application. In particular, with such widespread distribution of GABA throughout the brain, and given the many *different* receptor sites, modes of action and physiological effects, to add GABA throughout the entire central nervous system could have many and varied effects, not all healthy or safe. Does oral GABA survive digestion, remain stable in the circulation and get to the synapse in the first place? It is not known to be a circulating neurotransmitter. In any case, much more research is warranted before such intervention is justified.

(The vast scientific data pertaining to GABA receptors, which are of medical importance, are widely scattered throughout numerous heterogeneous Internet sources. That situation made the integrated acquisition of such data difficult and time consuming even for the Internet wizards. A novel server (GABA agent) is now available and freely accessible through the Internet, to assist in retrieving focused and integrated information related to GABA receptors from various public domain databases. This user friendly service may be accessed at the web address: http://www.ust.hk/gaba)

The 'scorched earth' approach just described for GABA is also reminiscent of the non-specific cancer therapies mentioned in Chapter

Four. In the twenty first century, good *science* demands that we do our homework to gain a better understanding of *nature*, so that applications and interventions can be targeted for efficacy and to minimize possible adverse effects.

Speaking of adverse effects, even the relatively safe benzodiazepines (as it was originally thought) turned out to have some.

Side Effects of Benzodiazepines

We do know that the benzodiazepines exert their therapeutic effects by enhancing the inhibitory neurotransmitter systems utilizing GABA. They bind to a specific site on the GABA receptor complex and act as receptor agonists (favoring the action of GABA per se). Valium has multiple active metabolites which increase the risk of "carryover" effects such as sedation and "hangover". More importantly, these drugs have the potential for producing drug **dependence** as we noted earlier. When patients stop using them, they show both physiological and behavioral symptoms which stimulate a craving for continual use and habituation. They are essentially addictive. People who discontinue benzodiazepines after taking them for a long time may experience rebound symptoms of sleep disturbance and anxiety, which can develop within hours or days after stopping the medication. Some patients have experienced the **withdrawal** symptoms including stomach distress, sweating and insomnia, that can last from one to three weeks. To make matters worse, Valium is short acting – with rapid absorption and peak blood concentrations in about one hour after ingestion. Shorter acting compounds have somewhat greater liability because of more rapid and abrupt onset of withdrawal symptoms. The systemic bioavailability is 100 percent and the half-life of valium in hours, by coincidence, is about equal to the user's age in years (as a Rule of Thumb).

The risk of physical dependence can be minimized by avoiding long term therapy – probably no more than about 6-8 weeks. Clinically, the anxiolytic indication for use is often not clear and a trial of therapy with a benzodiazepine is still reasonable. At the onset of such a trial, the desired therapeutic goal is best identified and the duration of therapy should be specified.

In addition to dependence and withdrawal symptoms, acute, sub-acute and chronic **tolerance** to benzodiazepines have been demonstrated in studies with both animals and humans. During long-term administration, tolerance commonly manifests itself as a decrease in side effects or a need to increase the dose to maintain symptomatic improvement.

The side effects most commonly reported with the use of benzodiazepines were drowsiness, fatigue and disturbances of gait. Many other adverse reactions have been observed but they are so infrequent that we can neglect them here. The frequency of side effects increases with age, dose, duration of therapy and also in cases of liver disease and low protein states.

Benzodiazepines have poor effects against the more particular anxiety conditions such as obsessive-compulsive disorder, panic disorder or post-traumatic stress disorder. These tend to be more effectively treated by the particular class of antidepressants we referred to earlier, the SSRI's. These warrant a brief discussion here.

ANTI-DEPRESSANTS

Most antidepressant drugs also have significant anti-anxiety and especially anti-panic effects in addition to their indicated anti-depressant actions. Many also have anti-obsessional effects. The tricyclic anti-depressants like imipramine have been used for the more particular anxiety disorders (e.g. panic disorder and obsessive-compulsive disorder), but the SSRI's like Prozac (Fluoxetine) have much more favorable tolerability and safety profiles, which have now made them the drugs of choice for these disorders (although higher cost is still an issue).

A word about the inhibitory neurotransmitter, serotonin. It is a small molecule related to the essential amino acid, tryptophan. In fact, serotonin is made by a relatively small number of cells in the brain starting with tryptophan. These cells are located in brainstem nuclei and from there, the neurons project axons to affect most areas of the brain. Since the discovery of serotonin in the 1950's, it has been intensely studied and it is clear that serotonergic neurons are implicated in mediating emotions and judgement, and much more. The key factor in both the effectiveness and safety profile of the SSRI's (selective serotonin re-uptake inhibitors) and their use as anti-depressants and more recently as anxiolytics, is the word *selective*. Serotonergic neurons have

such diverse influences in the central nervous system, that it is important to isolate the ones responsible for the desired clinical effects and not
practice (as we pointed out earlier) a 'scorched earth' policy in any
therapeutic intervention. SSRI's do just that, they effectively increase
local serotonin in the synapses of the *selective* neurons that lead to their
outstanding anti-depressant and anxiolytic effects while, as it were, ignoring by and large, all the other serotinergic activity in the central
nervous system. This critical principle is common in pharmacology;
one must know which are the special target sites of any given type for
any given drug. The body was not made for drugs, it is drugs that are
made for the body. Therefore the onus is on the scientist to tailor-make
each one with specificity.

SSRI's can cause agitation, nausea and sexual dysfunction.
Elderly people should take the lowest effective dose possible and those
with heart problems must be monitored closely.

Fluoxetine (Prozac) was recently shown to inhibit the binding
of GABA and flunitrazepam to the GABA(A) receptor complex in brain
cortical membranes. At low concentrations fluoxetine enhanced the
GABA-stimulated Cl⁻ ion uptake by a vesicular preparation from the
cerebral cortex of a rat. But at higher concentrations, fluoxetine did the
opposite – it inhibited the GABA-stimulated Cl⁻ uptake. The full significance is not clear but the interactions of this SSRI with the GABA(A)
receptor in some way, is at least consistent with its clinically observed
anxiolytic effect as well as its antidepressant effect.

One problem with antidepressants is the long delay before they
are fully effective – usually two to four weeks and sometimes up to
twelve weeks. People who take them can also experience a temporary
period of increased anxiety. As a result, about one third of patients stop
taking these antidepressants for anxiety disorders before the initial phase
of therapy has been completed.

Buspirone

In the mid-1980's, the FDA approved a new and promising
anxiolytic drug belonging to an entirely new class of azopyrines. The
generic product buspirone (known commercially as BuSpar™) is most
useful for the treatment of generalized anxiety disorder and is now frequently used as an adjunct to SSRI's like Prozac. It is a relatively

selective and partial, serotonin receptor agonist. Buspirone is believed to act as inhibitors to the presynaptic receptors. Unfortunately, it usually takes up to several weeks for the drug to be fully effective, and it is not very useful against panic attacks, OCD or PTSD. But unlike the benzodiazepines, buspirone is not addictive, even with long-term use, and it seems to have less pronounced side effects and no withdrawal effects, even when the drug is discontinued quickly. It therefore has a low potential for abuse and may be useful for adolescents and children. Some fairly common side effects include dizziness, drowsiness and nausea.

Other therapies

For completeness, we should at least mention that some patients can benefit from combining anxiolytic drug therapy with cognitive-behavioral therapy. The goal in the latter case is to help patients regain control of reactions to stress and stimuli, thus reducing the feeling of helplessness that often accompanies anxiety disorders. It helps the individual to understand the realities of an anxiety-provoking situation and to respond to reality with actions based on reasonable expectations. A variety of practical techniques have been used but it is fair to say that the benefits of multi modal therapies for anxiety need further study. Such combinations are certainly not always necessary and in fact, it would be appropriate and more cost-effective to reserve them for patients with more complex, complicated, severe or otherwise co-morbid disorders.

NATURAL ALTERNATIVES

Needless to say, because mental health is such a personal and in many ways, a subjective area, the scope for alternative interventions and unsubstantiated claims is both vast and attractive. The interest of the public and the wide range of natural products available has fostered the common exaggerated claims for beneficial, if not therapeutic, effects on mental health and illness. These include reports of enhanced memory in people taking the herbs Ginkgo or Ginseng, the use of the St. John's Wort flowers as an antidepressant, and for our purposes here, the use of the Kava root as an anxiolytic preparation.

We mentioned kava as one of the *herbs du jour* in Chapter One. It has been used as a popular tonic in the South Seas for centuries (perhaps millenia). With rising popularity in the U.S., it is said to alleviate stress, ease melancholy and generally elevate mood – all without addiction or hangover. Supermarkets, drugstores, health-food stores, discount chains, and now mail order and Internet companies have been stocking up and selling kava in capsules, droplets and tea bags.

The product is scientifically unproven but since 1996 a coalition of herbal product-makers devised an aggressive plan for marketing and promotion. Even the ABC TV network ran a story to suggest that kava might have the power to calm. And there are some anecdotal reports to suggest this. One of its best proponents is Dr. Hyla Cass, a UCLA psychiatrist no less, and co-author of a book on the subject; *Kava: Nature's Answer to Stress, Anxiety and Insomina* (Prima Health Publishers). The book speaks well for Kava, but it is all *nature*, **no hard science**. The prevailing suggestion is that kava contains an active ingredient in a class of molecules known as kava pyrones or kavalactones. These are plant metabolites that affect the limbic system we discussed earlier. It is, in part, an emotional center in the brain and does have regulatory functions. According to Dr. Cass, kava works on the same amino-acid sites as Valium. But while Valium binds to the GABA receptor complex sites to enhance the inhibiting neurotransmitter, kava it is believed , causes more of these sites to form. Those conclusions are suggested from studies with rats, and some German researchers have reported that kava is safe and effective for humans. It has since gained approval in Germany as a treatment for mild anxiety. That country's regulations in the area of alternative therapies are much more lenient than the U.S. FDA. For now, the FDA will allow kava manufacturers to promote their product only in a general way, advertising it as a supplement without citing any specific medical benefits.

To scientifically evaluate the role of kava and other natural or alternative treatments in mental health poses some major challenges. Too often, there is a lack of standardization and quality control. There are efforts being made to address this as we pointed out in Chapter One. New assays for kavalactones for example, are now standard in the industry. But there are issues of purity, bioavailability, amount and timing of dosages, and a number of other standardized practices common to the pharmaceutical industry. After all 'food supplements' are not held to the same standard as potentially lethal drug preparations.

In this author's judgement, it would be premature to arrive at any conclusions about the effective value of kava (or any other herbal preparation) as an established anxiolytic for widespread promotion. There have been very few studies to date to justify any such claims with certainty.

But there is some news to report. A new development based on good science offers the benefit of a new decapeptide derivative from a milk protein (casein) which we will show binds effectively to the GABA receptor, shows anxiolytic action in humans, and without the undesirable side effects seen with benzodiazepenes. This is the exciting subject of the next chapter.

Chapter Nine

NATURE'S
TRANQUILIZING PEPTIDE

Scientific discoveries come about in many different ways and cir cumstances. Some are found by *accident*, like Alexander Fleming discovery of penicillin; he went away and came back only to find that a mold on a petri dish that he inadvertently left standing, had opened up the era of antibiotics. Others came by spectacular *analysis* and insight like Einstein's Relativity which only the select few can still understand. The discovery by Gustavo Bounous of unique bioactive whey proteins containing essential precursors for the all-important glutathione modulation, illustrates a case of *serendipity* – looking for one thing and finding another. Watson and Crick discovered the double helix by adding one piece of data upon another until they solved the puzzle by *speculation*, and their gamesmanship opened the flood gates of molecular biology. Finally, some discoveries derive from *systematic inquiry*; it begins with a curious question which provokes experimental design, careful observation and then a cycle of investigation to find more and more answers. Such was the nature of the discovery that we are about to describe in this chapter.

A CURIOUS QUESTION

The discovery of nature's tranquilizing peptide originated a decade ago, with a question in the mind of Professor Guy Linden and Professor Jean-Francois Boudier, Ingredia, France and a research group at Nancy University, France. Having made the common observation of the calm state of a baby after drinking warm milk, the question arose if there was some ingredient in the milk or some product of digestion that had this calming (tranquilizing) effect on the little ones. It is not uncommon for babies to fall asleep on the breast while feeding. It is a restful experience for one reason or another and many a photographer has captured their facial expression, the countenance and temperament projected in skin tones and muscle relaxation, that only a content and tranquil baby can show.

Newborns are exposed to all kinds of aggression as soon as they leave the warm, secure, homeostatic environment of the womb. Just imagine what the experience of birth itself must be for the little fetus as it emerges into the world. The early Braxton-Hicks contractions must startle the mature and sensitive fetus. But it is only a sign of things to come, for soon tremor gives rise to turbulence, and turbulence to a tide and then a flood. Then the contracting pelvic walls make the darkness unbearable and so the innocent victim capitulates and starts to cooperate. But things go from bad to worse, as the intensity of the contracting walls increases to a crescendo, until the fetus loses all autonomy. The fragile life is pushed and pulled and catapulted beyond a point of no return, to emerge into the external world, hopefully screaming and desperate, but yet happy to have survived it all.

Then almost immediately upon arrival, something horrible starts to happen. The newborn baby comes face to face with the crushing realities of their new life. The obstetrician or pediatrician takes them up with those jaws she calls her hands and not infrequently, she smacks the little bottom just as it were, to set the tone for this new found existence. Little babies arrive tiny, immature and dependent. They are most vulnerable. So they cry. They make a mess and then they cry some more. Until … until they find their serenity latched on to a mother's breast and able to feed on nature's tranquilizing provision. No wonder they soon rest … so contentedly, so serenely, so joyfully. It is nature's way!

But environmental changes continue and the newborn is forced to contend with many forms of aggression, both physical and psychological. They are prone to anxiety, which initially must be a protective mechanism that alerts them to seek refuge, to cry for help, to root by reflex and then to feed. There, latched on to mother's breast, they take advantage of a route of escape from extreme anxiety. So, Professor Linden wondered, **is there some anxiolytic ingredient to be found in that natural provision we call milk?**

Moreover, it is known that the baby's enzymatic system is different from that of adults. Mature individuals have relatively high levels of the enzyme **pepsin**, the principal digestive enzyme of the stomach's (gastric) juice. It is formed from the precursor pepsinogen and hydrolyzes the peptide bond of proteins at low pH (high acid) values. It is particularly effective at breaking the peptide bonds adjacent to the amino acids phenylalanine and leucine, thereby converting macromolecular protein chains into smaller peptide molecules for absorption from the gastrointestinal tract.

Babies do not follow that course predominately. They digest proteins differently. They have low levels of the pepsin enzyme, but relatively high levels of a different enzyme called **trypsin**. Trypsin is also a proteolytic enzyme but it is formed in the small intestine from an inactive precursor provided by pancreatic secretions into the early part of the intestine (the duodenum). This precursor, trypsinogen, is converted into trypsin by the action of another enzyme called enterokinase, which is produced by the mucosal cells in the wall of the duodenum. Trypsin is a serine proteinase that hydrolyzes peptides, amides, esters etc. at bonds of the — COOH carboxyl groups of the amino acids arginine and lysine. This is the baby's preferred proteolytic enzyme. So, Dr. Linden asks again, **is there some link between the specific proteolytic enzyme trypsin, acting upon the proteins in milk to produce some derivative or adduct that could have this calming influence upon the baby?**

Isolating The Active Principle

The question posed by Professor Linden led to the design of systematic series of laboratory experiments. First, to choose a milk protein, hydrolyze it with trypsin and then separate the products so that each one could be tested for possible anxiolytic activity.

The major protein in milk we saw back in Chapter Two is casein. This is the milk protein which forms the predominant constituent of cheese. It is rather insoluble in water, but is soluble in dilute alkaline and salt solutions. Whole casein is obtained from milk by simple acid precipitation and neutralization using an alkali, by straightforward laboratory methods. Actually, whole casein is a collection of milk proteins which can be separated quite easily by a common laboratory and industrial process called chromatography. The main fractions that are eluted off a special DEAE-Cellulose column are respectively named beta-casein, kappa-casein, alpha-S1 casein and alpha-S2 casein. These fractions are well known and in particular, that of the selected alpha -S1 casein was already determined by others.

It is possible to prepare alpha-S1 casein in different ways:

One method is to fractionate whole casein on DEAE-cellulose as a stationary phase, using a discontinuous gradient of calcium chloride solution as the eluent. It has the advantage of fractionating all the caseins quickly. It may advantageously be implemented using in particular, DEAE Cellulose 52 as the anion exchange support. This material is a pre-swollen resin requiring no acid-base pre-treatment prior to first use.

Alternatively, it is possible to eliminate all caseins other than alpha-S1 casein in two steps only, while increasing the yield and the purity (>96%) of the alpha-S1 casein obtained. Thus, for example, it is possible to use a dry resin instead of a pre-swollen resin as before. By using a dry resin and omitting the pre-treatment required for obtaining a maximum load, the effectiveness of the load of the resin is limited, thereby limiting the fixation of the substrate.

University of Nancy researchers have developed their own method to isolate and to purify alpha –S1 casein by chromatography. Trypsin hydrolysis of this alpha-S1 casein was performed in buffered solution using bovine pancreatic trypsin as the enzyme.

The alpha-S1 casein hydrolysate obtained in this way, was subjected to two purification steps using two different columns in inverse phase high-performance liquid chromatography (HPLC).

With molecular separation techniques it was possible to isolate the peptides formed by the trypsin hydrolysis of alpha-S1 casein. These peptides were then used in *in vitro* tests to be described below, to test their effectiveness in binding to the benzodiazepine -type receptor. One specific peptide proved to be effective in this regard. It is a decapeptide with an amino acid sequence shown below, that represents the amino acids between positions 91 and 100 on the alpha-S1 casein chain.

We will heareafter refer to this as **'the Decapeptide'.**

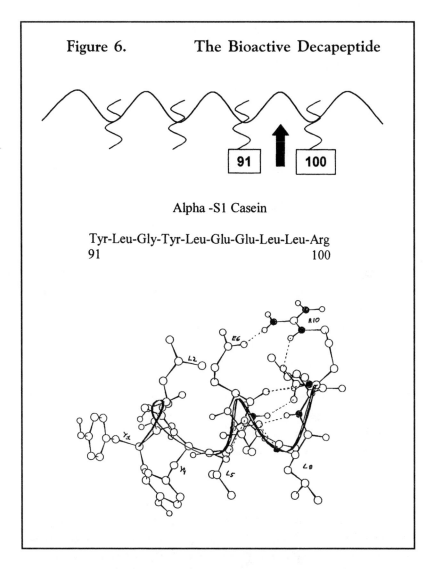

Figure 6.   The Bioactive Decapeptide

Alpha -S1 Casein

Tyr-Leu-Gly-Tyr-Leu-Glu-Glu-Leu-Leu-Arg
91   100

Knowing the active peptide sequence unequivocally, they were able to synthesize it by standard methods, and also to verify its bioactivity. The spatial structure of the Decapeptide was determined by a two dimensional method of nuclear magnetic resonance (NMR) spectroscopy, called circular dichroism, and by molecular dynamic simulation on computers (in collaboration with Professor Linden and a Nancy CNRS

Unit, France). They could then compare its specific binding with the known GABA(A) receptor using the spatial model from the Biosym Discover Program (San Diego , California).

The structure of the Decapeptide (as a time average) is shown in Figure 6. It adopts a 3(10) helical structure, initiated and terminated by an alpha-turn. It has rather interesting polar characteristics. The non-polar, oil- loving (hydrophobic) side chains are located on the same side of the molecule, while the more polar, water – loving (hydrophilic) side chains are located on the opposite side, giving the Decapeptide an amphiphilic characteristic. From this conformational study, the Decapeptide would be expected to cross different types of membranes (barriers). It is also interesting to observe that both the Decapeptide and the benzodiazepine nitrazepam were polyclosed, notably on a special length link.

It was already known that certain peptide fragments of the various caseins have various biological activities and in particular for the central nervous system, some have opiate and anti-opiate activities. These include the peptides 90-96, 90-95, 91-96 and 91-95 of alpha-S1 casein. Strangely enough, these are all smaller oligopeptides (smaller pieces, if you like) of the same bioactive Decapeptide 91-100 which was just identified as an effective but elusive ligand for the benzodiazepine receptor.

Other milk protein peptides have shown high biological activity as anti-hypertensive, mineral binding, immunomodulatory (as we saw in Chapter Five), and anti-thrombotic naturally-occurring moieties. Some of these additional gems from nature's goldmine will be illuminated at the end of this chapter.

A New Ligand for GABA(A)

The effectiveness of the Decapeptide in binding to the benzodiazepine receptor of the GABA receptor complex was demonstrated using a kit sold by Dupont (NENQUEST™, Drug Discovery System, NED—002). The method is based on competition between a radioactive ligand of the central benzodiazepine receptor and the molecule to be tested. If the molecule has an affinity for the receptor, it displaces the labeled ligand fixed to the receptor. Such displacement of the ligand as a function of the added concentration of the molecule to be tested, makes it possible to determine what is termed the **IC50** of the molecule. The

IC50 is the pharmacological concentration of the molecule which enables 50% of the maximum effect to be obtained. Therefore the lower the value of the IC50 for a given molecule being tested, the higher is the affinity of that molecule for the receptor.

The radioactive ligand used in this case was H-methyl-flunitrazepam, a benzodiazepine that possesses high specificity for the receptor (Ki = 1.2nM) and low non specific fixation. Commercial membrane preparations of central receptors of benzodiazepines were incubated with increasing concentrations of the sample to be tested and a fixed concentration of the radioligand. Incubation lasted one hour at +4°C. The temperature was deliberately chosen to be low, so as to limit association/dissociation between the receptor and the radio ligand. Flunitrazepam has a half-association time of 834 seconds at 0°C, and of 12 seconds at 35°C.   After one hour, the mixture was passed through a Whatman GF/E filter. Such filters retain the membranes and the ligands fixed to them (benzodiazepines and or peptide fragment(s) of alpha-S1 casein trypsin hydrolysate). After washing, the filters were placed in scintillation counter flasks containing a scintillation liquid. The emission of γ-rays from the remaining radioactive ligand was counted by a liquid scintillation counter.

As you would expect, if the tritium-labeled ligand has been displaced by the molecule under test, then a drop is observed in the level of radioactivity present on the filter.

In order to eliminate radioactivity due to a nonspecific bond between the tritium-labeled ligand and the receptor, a test was performed by incubating the membranes, the tritium-labeled ligand (at the same concentration as that used for the tests on a molecule whose IC50 is to be determined), and un-labeled flunitrazepam at an excess concentration of 500 times. The residual radioactivity was thus due only to nonspecific fixation, since it was assumed that all of the sites were occupied by un-labeled flunitrazepam.

A value B can be defined equal to the percentage of radioactivity fixed on the receptors for each concentration of the molecule under test, compared with a test performed using the membranes and the labeled flunitrazepam only (maximum radioactivity). It is possible to determine the IC50 of the molecule by plotting the base-10 loga-

rithm of B/(100-B) as a function of the base-10 logarithm of the concentration of the added molecule under test.

Remember we said above that the lower a value of IC50, the higher the affinity of the molecule for the receptor. For the Decapeptide purified by the inverse phase HPLC method described above, IC50 is about 88 μM. Similar activity was also found for fractions enriched with the Decapeptide in application of the other chromatographic methods outlined earlier.

These tests have also been performed using the Decapeptide obtained by peptide synthesis. It was found that the IC50 of the synthesized peptide was 370 μM. compared with 88 μM for the Decapeptide of natural origin. In other words, the synthetic Decapeptide showed a real but lower affinity for the benzodiazepine receptor.

We pointed out in the last chapter that the benzodiazepines were introduced in the 1960's to capitalize on the exploding market for drugs to help a public with real or imagined anxiety disorders. The first one Librium™, was never designed for a GABA receptor complex. The discovery of such an active site in synapses of the central nervous sytem came **after the fact**. Why this ancillary binding site exists functionally adjacent to the GABA(A) receptor site itself, even today is still not well understood. **Just imagine this: Here is a receptor for the most prevalent inhibitory neurotransmitter in the central nervous system – with one associated receptor site that becomes the receptor for the best selling drugs of all time and we still don't know what natural function it serves. At least, until now. But we do understand clearly the clinical benefits to be derived from using benzodiazepine-type ligands. They calm anxiety. They soothe a restless humanity.**

Maybe these French researchers were really on to something. Remember that this Decapeptide is a natural product derived from a protein found also in human breast milk, formed by hydrolysis with an enzyme uniquely elevated in babies. Is this all by nature's design? A unique receptor, a unique ligand, a unique effect. Isn't this *science* imitating *nature*?

Having demonstrated that this unique Decapeptide derived from common milk protein does bind effectively to the benzodiazepine receptor site, the question arose: what was the clinical effect to be observed with this new ligand? In search of answers, researchers turned to well-established animal models.

IN VIVO TESTS ON RATS

In the search for medicinal drugs, pre-clinical experiments with animals are obviously necessary to assess the safety and effectiveness of the compounds that are developed. Although it is virtually impossible to assess the subjective feelings and mental status of animals that are treated with drugs, animal research has clearly shown that the physiological effects of psychoactive drugs are almost always identical in animals and humans. Indeed, a drug's distribution in the CNS, its binding sites and receptors, its metabolism and elimination, the mechanisms of tolerance, and even the proportional effective dose are all highly correlated between animals and humans. These findings provide on-face validity that permits the results of animal tests to be applied to the understanding of the results of tests on humans.

Anxiolytic Activity

Anxiety is one of the few mental disorders for which excellent animal models have been developed. There are some 20-30 biobehavioral measures available to identify novel anxiolytic compounds and to predict their safety and efficacy. Researchers can reproduce some of the symptoms of human anxiety in animals by introducing different types of stressors, either physical or psychosocial.

The classic laboratory animal used for these studies is the **male Wistar Rat**, first "invented" at the Wistar Institute of Anatomy and Biology in Philadelphia. These rats were purposely bred in a quest for genetic homogeneity and were the first animals 'standardized' for use in laboratory research. They comprise a classic inbred albino as well as numerous other strains maintained through controlled breeding and husbandry dating back many years. Early Wistar rats constitute a major portion of the laboratory rat gene pool. Their descendants and namesakes are still used in laboratories throughout the world. They are the equivalent in animal research, if you like, to pure chemicals in chemistry research, which allows the control of many otherwise genetic variables. Again, this illustrates the power of *science* in union with *nature*.

Pre-clinical studies on male Wistar Rats were carried out by researchers in France led by Mr. Messaoudi as Scientific Director and with Professor Desor as Scientific Advisor and Quality Insurance Auditor. To measure anxiety in the rat, the French researchers used two different but well established animal models observing the behavioral responses of the Male Wistar Rat.

Procedure.   The first one was the **Elevated Plus-Maze Test** described in 1985 by Pellow and colleagues. It is based on the tendency of the rat to avoid new environments or exposures. The animal shows a morbid aversion to or dread of novelty for the unknown – a characteristic technically termed neophobia (Gk.*neo* – new, *phobos* – fear). The rat is observed by hidden video cameras for convenient observation and replay, exploring a cross-shaped maze with different arms or branches, some open and some closed. The plus-maze had four branches that were 50cm long and 10cm wide. The two closed branches were surrounded by walls that were 25cm high (the top being left open for observation) and the entire maze was 50 cm above the ground. The center of the maze communicated with the two open arms and the two closed arms. The principle is rather simple: the rodents have a natural fear of heights and open spaces. In dim light the more anxious the rat, the less the rat will tend to explore the open arms, which does not correspond to natural behavior.

The number of times the animal enters the open arms, the closed arms, and the total number of times the rat enters the arms are important parameters. The time passed in each type of branch was also measured. Other parameters (a total of 22) such as the number of times the rat stood up, the number of times it groomed itself (signs of anxiety), or latency of first entry into an open or closed branch and so on, were taken into account. The animal was observed for 5 minutes after being placed in the center of the apparatus. Its entire behavior was filmed to avoid errors.

All trials were double-blind tested as we outlined in Chapter Three. Observations were performed on a control group of 20 rats (CTR), on a positive control group comprising 20 rats that received diazepam (DZP), and on a group of 20 rats that were treated with trypsin hydrolysate of alpha-S1 casein (HT). The control group (CTR) received an intraperitoneal injection of solvent only, which was a mixture of gelatin and mannitol (0.5%/5%) dissolved in water. The mixture serves to place diazepam into suspension, given that diazepam is insoluble in conventional injectable solvents (water, normal saline, ethanol 10%). The animals in all the groups were injected half an hour before going to the plus-maze. To begin the experiments, each rat was placed in the center of the apparatus.

Results. The results are given in Figures 7, 8, and 9, which show, as a function of the type of treatment: the percentage of entries into open branches (Figure 7); the number of entries into open branches (BO)) and into closed branches (BF), (Figure 8); and the time spent in the open branches (Figure 9).

It can be concluded that in this test, and studying major parameters only, trypsin hydrolysate of alpha-S1 casein had an action comparable to that of diazepam but with a smaller quantitative effect; this is not surprising since only the crude hydrolysate was used.

Figure 7.

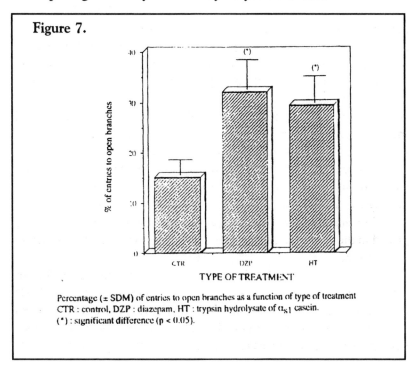

Percentage ($\pm$ SDM) of entries to open branches as a function of type of treatment
CTR : control, DZP : diazepam, HT : trypsin hydrolysate of α_{S1} casein.
(*) : significant difference ($p < 0.05$).

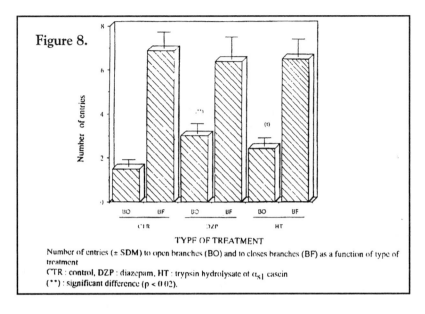

Figure 8.

Number of entries (± SDM) to open branches (BO) and to closes branches (BF) as a function of type of treatment

CTR : control, DZP : diazepam, HT : trypsin hydrolysate of α_{S1} casein

(**) : significant difference (p < 0.02).

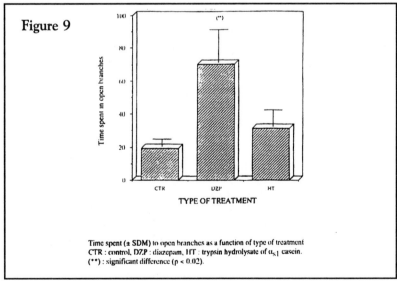

Figure 9

Time spent (± SDM) to open branches as a function of type of treatment
CTR : control, DZP : diazepam, HT : trypsin hydrolysate of α_{S1} casein.
(**) : significant difference (p < 0.02).

The second model used by the French resesearchers for studying anxiety in the rat was the **Conditioned Defensive Burying Test** described by Treit and Pinel (1981).

Procedure. In this case, the apparatus consisted of a rectangular chamber with an electrical shock probe extending in from one of the walls. The floor of the chamber is lined with a bedding of saw dust. Once the rat was placed in the chamber, a number of behaviors were observed and recorded. When the probe was charged to threaten the rat, it quickly would retreat to the back of the cage away from the probe, while facing it, and it would start to push the bedding toward the probe using its snout and forepaws. This was its defensive burying (DB) action, an act of apparent self-preservation in the face of imminent danger – a sign of true anxiety –type behavior. Therefore, one would measure the duration of each DB response, the number of DB responses or head stretches towards the probe, and the percentage of approaches towards the probe, followed by retreats.

Results:

Both the alpha-S1 casein trypsin hydrolysate (Prodiet F200) and the isolated Decapeptide active ingredient, showed definite anxiolytic-like activity in the male Wistar rat.

The effect is similar when administered either orally or intraperitoneally. This well-established animal model is a good indicator for the clinical significance of such a pharmacological intervention. This is consistent with the *in vitro* observation that the Decapeptide binds to the benzodiazepine receptor site of the GABA(A) receptor complex, shown earlier by displacement of a radioactive benzodiazepine ligand.

A new question arises soon after observing any pharmacological action: it may be effective, yes, but is it safe? Are there any unwanted side effects to offset any potential clinical benefit?

No Side Effects

As we pointed out in the last chapter, the introduction of the benzodiazepines in the 1960's was a mixed blessing. Those drugs, particularly Valium, took the market by storm. For several years, there was a high demand from both patients and physicians and clearly, this must reflect not only their high efficacy but also a fairly good safety profile with few side effects. However, it became apparent whenever patients tried to discontinue these drugs, that there were problems related to dependence and withdrawal. Other major side effects generally attributed to benzodiazapines included tolerance and some degree of memory loss.

Thus, it is not surprising that the researchers focused initially on these potential side effects of the new bioactive Decapeptide and the unfractionated alpha-S1 trypsin hydrolysate (Prodiet F200). However, even before this, there are some standard behavioral tests, called collectively the Irwin Test, which are usually done to look for potential side effects for a typical drug acting on the central nervous system.

1. Behavioral Effects: Irwin Test

Procedure

Decapeptide solutions were prepared just prior to their intraperitoneal administration to the Wistar rats at 2:00p.m. The animals were then observed in comparison with other 'control' rats which were given saline as placebo. Observations were performed 30, 60 and 120 minutes after administering the peptide and also 24 hours later for possible delayed death.

Observed Variables

The following items concerning behavioral changes, but also physiological and toxic symptoms, and mortality were recorded:

- *Behavior:*
  - *spontaneous activity;*
  - *affective motor response;*
  - *sensorimotor response.*
- *Neurology:*
  - *posture;*
  - *muscle tone;*
  - *equilibrium and gait;*
  - *CNS excitement.*
- *Autonomic NS:*
  - *eyes;*
  - *secretions and excretions;*
  - *miscellaneous*
- *Toxicology:*
  - *mortality*

Results:

In the experimental conditions, the characteristics of the Decapeptide that appeared were all in favor of an anti-stress profile.

The safety profile was satisfactory. There was no modification in behavior, neurology, autonomic nervous system and toxicology.

2. Major Side Effects Tested

a) NO DEPENDENCE

The Decapeptide was double-blind tested for its possible addictive effect using the standard paradigm of Conditioned Place Preference in the male Wistar rats, described below. Diazepam was used as a reference substance. Conditioned place preference was defined as a positive difference in the time spent on the unconditioned stimulus-associated side between post-and pre-conditioning tests.

Experimental Device: *The experimental apparatus consisted of a rectangular box (50 x 25 x 40 cm) divided into two compartments separated by an overhead door. The compartments are characterized by the color of the walls and the texture of the floors: black walls with smooth floors versus gray walls with corrugated floors. The rats could then distinguish between the contrasted environmental conditions in the two compartments.*

Procedure: *The test was performed in blind conditions and the recorded behaviors were scored by experimenters unaware of the administered products. Session 1: This session was carried out over 3 days, 15 minutes per day, in order to familiarize the rats with the apparatus. The animal was allowed to move freely between compartments. On the third day, each rat's preference for one of the two compartments was determined (that is, the compartment where the rat spent the most time). Session II: On days 4, 6, 8 and 10, rats were treated with the tested compound and enclosed individually into their initial non-preferred compartment for 45 minutes. On alternate days, each rat received a saline solution injection and was enclosed individually into the initial preferred compartment for 45 minutes. Session III: On the 12th day, the addition test was carried out: the rats were placed indi-*

vidually between the compartments for 15 minutes with access to both compartments. The time spent in each compartment was measured.

SESSIONS I AND III were monitored and recorded on VHS-videotape.

Results: Rats treated with Saline and the Decapeptide spent the same time in the non-preferred compartment. In contrast, Diazepam-treated rats spent significantly increased time in the non-preferred compartment and significantly increased their number of crossings between the two compartments after pre-conditioning tests. One could then draw the following bottom-line conclusion:

Unlike Diazepam, the Decapeptide did not induce conditioned place preference in the male Wistar rat.

b) NO MEMORY LOSS

The Decapeptide was double-blind tested for its possible amnesic effect on social memory in the male Wistar rat by another standardized procedure described below. Diazepam was used as a reference substance. The rather unusual studied variable here was the change in the investigation duration of the juvenile's ano-genital area by the adult rat on the second exposure when compared to the first exposure.

Procedure: *Three days prior to the memory test, the rats were isolated in individual cages. On the test day, all rats under investigation were placed in a dim lit experimental room and remained there for 2 hours prior to the start of the first exposure. Observations were carried out with a video camera. All rats were tested in their home cage and each test consisted of 5 minute exposure to a juvenile, followed by a second exposure to the same juvenile at 30-minute intervals. Between the two successive presentations, juveniles were individually kept in small boxes.*

The products were given to the rats immediately after the first exposure to the juvenile stimulus. Investigation was defined as direct contact (nosing, sniffing) of the juveniles ano-genital area by the adult rat for 5 minutes. The test was performed and the recorded behaviors were recorded by experimenters unaware of the administered products.

Results: During the first minute of the test, as well as during the 5 minute test session, the duration of investigations by the adult rats, treated with either saline or the Decapeptide, significantly decreased on the second exposure when compared to the first exposure. In contrast to this, the adult rats treated with Diazepam spent as much time or significantly increased time investigating the juvenile on the second exposure, when compared to the first exposure. One could justifiably draw the following bottom-line conclusion:

Unlike Diazepam, the Decapeptide did not show any amnesic effect on social memory in the male Wistar rat.

c) NO TOLERANCE
The Conditioned Defensive Burying Test described earlier was used to assess the phenomenon of tolerance to the alpha-S1 casein trypsin hydrolysate (Prodiet F200) in the male Wistar rat after chronic administration (4 days).

Unlike Diazepam, no similar tolerance to the Prodiet F200 was apparent when the product was administered twice daily for the same period, well above that used to demonstrate positive anxiolytic activity.

Summary: The efficacy of the alpha-S1 casein trypsin hydrolysate (Prodiet F200) and the isolated bioactive Decapeptide have both been shown earlier to have positive anxiolytic activity by binding to the benzodiazepine receptor of the GABA(A) receptor complex. All the results just described demonstrate a clear picture of safety for this new *natural* anxiolytic when administered to the male Wistar rat. The appropriate, well-established animal models show none of the same adverse effects as demonstrated by diazepam (Valium) administered under similar conditions. In particular, there was no dependence, no memory loss and no tolerance effect observed.

This set the stage for human trials which will be discussed next.

HUMAN TRIALS

As a result of the pre-clinical studies in animals, it was shown that the unfractionated alpha-S1 casein trypsin hydrolysate (Prodiet F200) and the isolated bioactive Decapeptide had similar positive anxiolytic activity (at different dosage levels) and neither showed any significant side effects. It was therefore decided to perform clinical studies in humans, using the hydrolysate Prodiet F200 .

Two studies received the authorization and the agreement of the French Health Authorities to be performed by registered clinical units. These studies were sponsored by Ingredia with Professor Jean-Francois Boudier as Scientific Director.

These studies were unicenter, comparative and double-blind. The selection procedure involved a screening of the volunteers with a complete clinical and biological examination including EKG. There were strict inclusion and exclusion criteria

Twenty four (24) volunteers were included in the first study and forty two (42) volunteers were included in the second study.

We will describe each of these two clinical trials in turn.

A.   First Clinical Trial
1.1   Study Objective

It is of interest to perform a study in humans aimed at evaluating the possible anxiolytic effect of the Prodiet F200 hydrolysate through several standard parameters. The objective was to evaluate the consequences of the milk protein hydrolysate (Prodiet F200) ingestion by healthy human volunteers on their hemodynamic parameters (blood pressure, heart rate), anxiety and cognitive function, under conditions of moderate stress.

1.2   Psychometric Tests Used

The immediate goal here was to evaluate anxiety evolution, in a moderate stress situation, after or without 15 days of Prodiet F200 consumption. Two appropriate and standardized anxiety scales were used:

1. **Cattell Anxiety Scale** – this provides a measure of the general level of anxiety; it requires completion of a 15 minute questionnaire.

2. **Speilberger Anxiety Inventory State-Level** including two

sub-scales (each with a 15 minute questionnaire).
- Anxiety-state scale – this provides a sensitive, transient, modification indicator for anxiety induced by a stress situation;
- Anxiety-level scale, evaluating anxiety as a stable disposition.

There is a relation between the second anxiety-level scale and the Cattell scale, since these two scales can be considered as equivalent measures of anxiety, seen as a stable disposition in the subjects. It means the subjects' natural state of anxiety before product ingestion.

The Spielberger anxiety-state scale allows appreciation of the anxiety–linked modifications in this study in reference to the test situation sessions, assuming that those test achievements induce a moderate stress. The *acute* stress situation was induced by performing different attention tests in restrictive time:

- Attention/Concentration Test: numbers to tick in 10 minutes
- Mental Rapidity Test (Pacaud test) in 8 minutes
- Stroop Test in 3 minutes

These three tests are commonly used to evaluate cognitive functions, especially the subjects' attention skills, before and after the product ingestion period. They have been previously validated by others on important populations. The achievement of these tests was a practical way of inducing stress and the results obtained provided a stress-resistance level, in terms of attention.

1.3 Conclusion

After the stress test, human volunteers with a high anxiety level as a stable disposition had a slower increase on their global anxiety-state score when they received the milk protein hydrolyzate (Prodiet F200) by oral administration, compared to placebo controls. (Fig.10)

There was no apparent effect of Prodiet F200 on cognitive function or on hemodynamic parameters under these conditions.

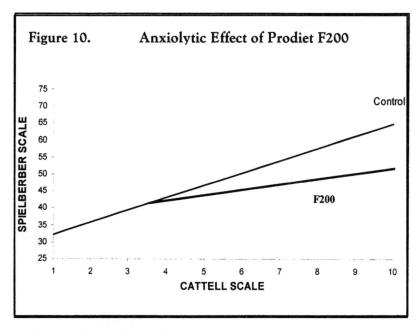

Figure 10.   Anxiolytic Effect of Prodiet F200

B. Second Clinical Trial
2.1   Study Objective
The objective of this second study was similar to the first. It was to evaluate again the consequences of the milk protein hydrolysate (Prodiet F200) ingestion by a statistical group of healthy volunteers on their hemodynamic parameters (blood pressure) and hormonal stress indicators (cortisol and ACTH) under conditions of moderate stress. However, there were several important differences when compared to the previous clinical trial.

2.2   Psychometric Tests Used
In this study, anxiety was measured with two different types of testing during test sessions: **The Cold Pressor Test** is classified among the *physical provocation* type of tests, in comparison with the other types of tests (eg. *psychological* type of tests like **the Stroop test** which was also used). In practice, for this Cold Pressor test, the volunteers put their hand into cold water (at 2°C), which induces a sympathetic nervous activation, close to the ache, but this reaction is the same as previously observed with other stress causes. In principle, the volunteers

could each react differently against the 2 stress tests: physical and psychological. Also, 2 different volunteers could react at different levels during the 2 tests. The idea was that by differentiating the anxiety tests, it should be possible to explain or approach the possible reaction mechanism of the bioactive Decapeptide. Both The Cold Pressor test and/or the Stroop test are frequently used to check anxiety activity, and they have been shown to be perfectly reproducible. This is just good basic science.

2.3 RESULTS

During the Stroop test, blood pressure increased significantly lower ($p<0.03$) in volunteers receiving Prodiet F200.

During the Cold Pressor test, the blood cortisol level remained stable in the control group receiving placebo (no significant level of change), while it decreased significantly ($p< 0.005$) in the group receiving Prodiet F200. Cortisol is a stress hormone released by the adrenal cortex. The cortisol level is a stress indicator.

During the stress tests (Stroop test and Cold Pressor test), adrenocorticotropic hormone (ACTH) levels in the blood, increased in the control group ($p< 0.09$) and **not** in the group receiving Prodiet F200 (Fig. 11). ACTH is a normal product of the anterior pituitary gland and acts as a controller of the secretion of the adrenal hormone, cortisol. ACTH level is therefore another stress indicator.

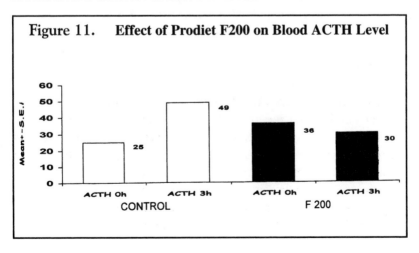

Figure 11. Effect of Prodiet F200 on Blood ACTH Level

Conclusions

These results clearly demonstrate the efficiency of the milk protein hydrolysate (Prodiet F200) as an anxiolytic in healthy human volunteers. Both physical and psychologic stress tests consistently showed that the changes in the group receiving Prodiet F200, compared to the control group receiving placebo, reflect a dulling of the anxiety response upon exposure to these stressors.

These results in healthy human volunteers are entirely consistent with what is to be expected from the earlier studies *in vitro* and in rats. Those studies unambiguously demonstrated the affinity of the bioactive Decapeptide ingredient for the benzodiazepine-type receptor site of the GABA(A) receptor complex. This agonist effect enhances the inhibiting action of the neurotransmitter GABA and so modulates the anxiety response. Furthermore, in contrast to the known side-effects of benzodiazepines, the Prodiet F200 showed no similar side-effects and are indicative of a more safe and tolerable clinical profile. Again, this is not surprising considering firstly, that it is derived from a protein endogenous to breast milk (just as it is in cow's milk too) and secondly, that it is a product of trypsin enzymatic action, that enzyme being the predominant enzyme for proteolysis in newborns. Since newborns are exposed to all types of aggression and are therefore prone to anxiety, this would appear to be a natural defensive system with a purpose.

Recall that enigma we pointed out in the last chapter. A common important (GABA) receptor in the CNS - with an associated receptor suitable for (benzodiazepine –type) *drugs* but no natural ligands identified until now? Now that we know of this bioactive Decapeptide - **Could it be that this is a major reason why the benzodiazepine-type receptor is there *naturally* in that location in the brain, in the first place?**

Think about it. First, there are the cysteine precursors - discovered in **nature's goldmine** - that effectively get into the human cell and modulate glutathione production. That in itself, proposes to impact the *glutathione revolution* and prompt a novel prospective as we re-think medicine and health in the Wellness Age. Now we find, also in **nature's goldmine**, a unique Decapeptide that is active in the major inhibitory GABA- chloride ion receptor complex in the brain. This too is central to the most common mental condition in modern society – anxiety. These are miracle ingredients indeed.

Once again, Nature preceded Science!

PNT   200

With the track record of the drugs having anxiolytic activity in the North American market – from Miltown, to Librium and Valium, to Prozac – the discovery of a milk protein hydrolyzate that was proven by good science to have similar anxiolytic activity and without side effects, there was clear potential for commercialization of such a product. So the originators moved to gain patent protection for their discovery and were successful in obtaining a method-of-use patent based on this research.

U.S. Patent 5,846,939
Date of Patent: December 8, 1998
Use of a Decapeptide with benzodiazepine-type activity for preparing medicines and food supplements.
Abstract:
        The present invention relates to the use of the Decapeptide having the amino acid sequence SEQ ID NO: 1 ## STR 1 ## in the preparation of medicines having benzodiazepine-type activity, particularly useful for the treatment of convulsions and anxiety. The invention also relates to pharmaceutical compositions, food supplements and food stuffs for special diets containing the said Decapeptide.
Assigned to: Société Coopérative Laitiere d`Artois et des Flandres, La Prosperite Fermiere (Arras, France)

Original patent: France, Number 94 14362. La Prosperite Fermiere is the parent company of INGREDIA .

The additional claim that the Decapeptide may be 'useful for the treatment of convulsions' is consistent with well-known benzodiazepine-type activity and derives from additional *in vivo* studies in rats not detailed in this book. Those results demonstrated that when seizures in the animal were induced by injecting pentylenetetrazol (a molecule acting to block chloride channels of the GABA receptor complex, to produce symptoms like epileptic seizure), the induced seizures were weaker, delayed and of shorter duration when the Prodiet F200 hydrolysate was previously injected. Thus, the Prodiet F200 clearly had a protective (anti-convulsant) effect in these animals.

The product has since been commercialized and is marketed in North America through Immunotec Research Ltd, – a leader in twenty first century milk – derived technology. The original naturally-sourced product has the registered trademark PNT 200 (peptide natural tranquil, 200+ mg) It is unique and with a patent protecting its method-of-use, there is nothing else like it currently available on the market. The milk from which it is made comes from dairy herds in France and Switzerland that are pesticide free, antibiotic free and free of growth hormones. It is packaged under license in Quebec, Canada under the strictest pharmaceutical grade conditions.

PNT 200 is indicated as an OTC (over the counter) preparation for the relief of occasional simple nervous tension, nervousness due to common overwork and fatigue, for calming down and relaxing, for resolving irritability, or for occasional difficulty in falling asleep due to restless anxiety. Its effect is to aid relaxation, to relieve the symptoms of stress and frustration, and to relieve occasional sleeplessness.

PNT 200 is contraindicated with the simultaneous use of alcohol or drugs prescribed for mental illness (acting on the central nervous system); or during pregnancy or lactation; or during demanding or hazardous activity such as operating heavy machinery or long distance driving. That is only prudent.

Now, there's even more yet to be gained from exploring any other rich gems that nature may have buried in the goldmine. Clearly, there's something there for you.

OTHER PEPTIDE GEMS

We have now seen two extraordinary examples of the bioactive peptides that are present in the amino acid sequences of milk proteins:

(a)   The bioactive Decapeptide that binds to the benzodiazepine-
        type ligand of the GABA-receptor complex, and
(b)   the cysteine-containing dimers in whey proteins that enter hu-
        man cells to up-regulate glutathione synthesis for cell protec
        tion and immune modulation.

These are indeed but two gems in nature's goldmine. There are many
more which are less well characterized but which offer much promise as
true nutraceuticals.

According to DeFelice (1995), a 'nutraceutical' is *any substance
that is a food or part of a food that provides medical or health benefits,
including prevention and treatment of disease.* It is not surprising that
nature's goldmine - the nutritional link between generations - should be
abounding in such nutraceuticals. After all, it is the best that nature has
to offer for species propagation and survival. Different mammalian
species share many of the same physiological needs and many of the
gems in nature's goldmine are found to be common among different
species.

Many, but not all, of the bioactivities of milk are attributable to
the proteins and peptides either present in the mammary secretions, or
derived (released) by the action of proteolytic enzymes, during gastrointestinal digestion, for example, or during food processing. Although
other animal and even plant proteins contain potential bioactive sequences, milk proteins now represent the principal source of the wide
range of biologically active peptides.

These bioactive peptides, as we have seen for the anxiolytic
Decapetide above, can be produced by any of the three potential processes:

1.   *In vivo* gastrointestinal digestion of the
        appropriate precursor proteins;
2.   *In vitro* proteolysis with enzymes on a
        laboratory scale; or
3.   Chemical synthesis from amino acids.

In either case, thanks to modern science, it is now practical to
harness the individual ingredients from nature's goldmine and to chara-

cterize and study the particular physiological effects of each component gem, to exploit potential applications for health and even medicine.

In the last quarter century, research has proliferated on these bioactive peptides and the accumulating data points to their important physiological effects and the prospects for both nutraceutical and even pharmaceutical applications. Recent reviews (1998) have been published by Meisel, (Germany), Torne and Debabbi (France), and Schanbacher and co-workers (USA), among others.

Here we will only summarize some key observations to underscore the richness of nature's goldmine that might even justify one reviewers concluding metaphor. Nature's goldmine (milk) is *"the mammalian mother's original pharmacopea, optimized for the infants of each mammalian species"*. It goes beyond the mere nutritional value as a source of amino acids for protein synthesis. It provides in these bioactive peptides, novel means for modulating a variety of important regulatory processes in the body.

We will therefore take a brief look into the following areas:

(i)   opiod activity as it pertains to gut motility and function in the central   nervous system;
(ii)   the inhibition of an important enzyme for regulating blood pressure locally;
(iii)   mineral-binding proteins and peptides;
(iv)   immune modulating peptides;
(v)   infection fighters; and
(vi)   anti-clotting factors

Opioid activity

The opium poppy has been used in Asia Minor and Southeastern Europe for over two thousand years. Its juice was known to contain an agent which relieved pain, produced sleep or drowsiness, relieved diarrhea, and in low doses, produced a blissful or euphoric state. The first active ingredient was isolated and purified in the early nineteenth century -- it was the prototype "opiate" called morphine (after *Morpheus*, the Greek god of sleep). The term "opioid" was later introduced to include substances not derived from opium. By 1973, stereo specific receptors for opioid drugs were proven to exist in the central nervous

system. Two years later, endogenous opioids were found and characterized as short-chain peptides (enkephalins) and soon, longer peptides
(endorphins) were discovered.

Opioid receptors fall into different classes and types and it is
sufficient here only to point out that some of these are found in the
nerves controlling the tone and motility of the small intestine and other
peripheral tissues. When activated, there is a marked reduction in the
propulsive peristaltic movement, resulting in constipation and/or an anti-
diarrheal effect. Stimulation of receptors in the chemoreceptor trigger
zone in the brain can also lead to nausea and vomiting at the other end.

Opiod peptides derived from milk casein are called casomorphins
or exorphins. They can bind to opioid receptors on the cells that line the
intestinal wall. Those derived from Beta-casein are the most potent.
Others are derived from alpha–S1-casein, beta-lactoglobulin and alpha-lactalbumin. These can all be derived *in vitro* but only the beta-
casomorphin has been shown to be present after *in vivo* digestion of
milk in calves, and not in humans. The net effect of casomorphins is to
inhibit the rate of gastric emptying and intestinal motility. This can
modulate the passage of digested foods and therefore absorption of important nutrients.

Beta-casormorphin has been found in the blood and cerebrospinal fluid of pregnant and lactating women.

Opioid antagonists have been found in kappa-casein from cow's
milk and human milk, and also in human lactoferrin.

Blood pressure activity

There are several different physiological mechanisms that determine and control blood pressure. The important renin-angiotensin
system has been the focus of different pharmaceutical approaches to
controlling hypertension. The angiotensins are peptides derived from a
plasma globulin. Angiotensin I is a decapeptide formed by the action of
the enzyme renin released by the kidneys. A second enzyme called an-
giotensin-converting-enzyme (ACE) converts angiotensin I into a very
powerful vasoconetrictor called angiotensin II. ACE inhibitors are widely
used as antihypertensive agents (for blood pressure control).

The enzyme ACE has many functions and is located in different
tissues. It plays a key role in regulating local levels of several

endogenous bioactive peptides, among which are the casokinins from human and bovine casein. Highly active casokinins are the bovine alpha-S1-casein sequence of amino acids in positions 23-27, and the beta-casein sequence 177-183. The structures of the ACE inhibitory peptides show some common features - suggestions of a structure - activity relationship. There is much on-going research in this area to elucidate the precise mechanisms of action.

The net effect may be to reduce hypertension and increase local blood flow, especially in the intestinal mucosa or mammary epithelium (breast linings).

Mineral building

Much of the phosphorus found in milk is bound to casein, and in such a way that the casein phosphopeptides contain a unique cluster of phosphate and glutamyl residues with negatively charged side-chains that create a novel binding site for positive mineral ions, especially calcium. These soluble organo-phosphate salts may function as efficient carriers for minerals and could therefore exert an influence on the absorption of calcium and other minerals and trace elements from the intestine. In addition, the calcium-binding phosphopeptides have been shown to have an anticariogenic effect. They protect against dental caries by recalcification of the dental enamel.

Other proteins - including lactoferrin, vitamin B_{12}-binding protein, folate binding protein, beta-lactoglobulin and alpha-lactalbumin - are assumed to interact with either minerals, vitamins or nutrients by a specific mechanism to affect their absorption. Lactoferrin, in particular, has been examined for iron transport.

Immune modulation

Both *in vitro* and *in vivo* studies have demonstrated that the bioactivity of several immunopeptides is unrelated to the glutathione modulation mechanisms of cell-defense described in some detail in Part 2 of this book. Immunopeptides derived from casein for example, such as residues 194-199 of alpha-S1-casein and residues 63-68 or 191-193 of beta-casein, stimulate the phagocytosis of sheep red blood cells by macrophage cells from the peritoneum of mice. These also exert a protective effect against *Klebsiella pneumoniae* infection in mice after in travenous injection.

The precise mechanism by which these immunopeptides act is not yet clear. It is tempting to associate the opioid action with the immuno-modulatory effects, since opioid receptors are present on T-lympho-cytes and human phagocytic white blood cells. In addition, both mac-rophages and lymphocytes express receptors for many biologically ac-tive mediators. But we must not yield to temptation when that is all there is. Science only *begins* with asking the question. The answers need to be pursued further.

Infection fighters

Some antimicrobial peptides have been derived from the whey protein lactoferrin. This protein plays an important role in host defense in different ways. We saw in Chapter Five that it was a key source of bioactive cysteine, the rate-limiting precursor for glutathione synthesis. It is also an obvious carrier for iron which transports oxygen.

More particularly though, the peptide fragment with residues 17-41, has been generated *in vitro* by pepsin cleavange. It contains an intramolecular disulfide bond and has bactericidal properties more po-tent than lactoferrin. Perhaps because it is smaller, the peptide called lactoferricin can get to more confined target sites on the microbial sur-face. The lactoferricin structure shows clusters of positive charges that may kill sensitive microrganisms by increasing cell-membrane perme-ability.

Recent studies also show antibacterial activity for an alpha-S2-casein peptide, residues 165-203, with a similar structure. It inhibits the growth of *E-coli* and *Staph . carnosus*.

Clotting activity

The clotting of blood and milk apparently show a number of similarities at the molecular level. The interacting region of the fibrino-gen gamma-chain (protein) in platelet aggregation is the C-terminal resi-due of twelve amino acids, a sequence which itself possesses similar inhibitory effects as some fragments produced from trypsin proteolysis of bovine kappa-casein. These casoplatelins are peptides also derived from the C-terminal part of the kappa-casein. They inhibit the aggrega-tion of ADP-activated platelets as well as binding of human fibrinogen gamma-chain to the specific receptor site on the surface of platelets. They include sequences of residues 106-116, 106-112, 112-116 and 113-116 - the main antithrombotic peptides dervied from kappa-casein.

It is important to emphasize again that even if some bioactive peptides are not released *in vivo* under normal physiological conditions, it is possible in principle, to harness their beneficial health or medical effects where indicated, through commercial production by modern technology. Nature's goldmine is indeed rich and waiting to be further exploited in the service of man.

We are still perhaps, merely scratching the surface. But we should proceed with caution, justifying every indication for any possible dietary supplementation or in the extreme, pharmaceutical preparation.

We need lots more data.

PART

4

TAKING
HOME
GOLD!

Chapter Ten

THINK CALCIUM: THINK MILK?

We have now seen that *buried* beneath all the advertising and promotion of milk and dairy products, are some real unique, nutritional nuggets that become ever so precious when exploited by science and technology. Considering the central role of glutathione in the defense of individual cells, who would have looked to common whey proteins for a particular bioactive conformation that would deliver the rate-limiting precursor inside the living cell, for modulation of the entire immune system? Or who would imagine that a natural product of milk protein digestion would find an affinity for a special receptor adjacent to the active gateway of the most common and predominant inhibitory neurotransmitter in the central nervous system? There we have found, are real gems from nature's goldmine.

But ask the average consumer about milk and inevitably the first (if not often, the only) benefit to be identified clearly is the availability of calcium. That's the same calcium that everyone knows will make strong bones and healthy teeth. It legitimizes the intense promotion of milk for children in schools, often for patients in hospitals, for the expectant and nursing mothers, for the fragile seniors ... and for everyone it seems. Let them drink of nature's goodness to derive all its benefits – but especially the calcium. Why?

CALCIUM IN THE BODY

Calcium is the most abundant mineral in the human body. To give you an idea of how much calcium there is, consider that the body of a typical young adult male has about 2.6lbs (1.2kg) of element calcium. Most of that, about 99% in fact, is in the bones and teeth, where it plays essentially a structural role. That accounts for the strong bones and teeth that everyone talks about. The remaining 1% is present in body tissues and fluids where it is essential for cell metabolism, muscle contraction and nerve impulse transmission. But none of this is static. There is continuous exchange of calcium between the skeleton and blood and other parts of the body. If the bones were the central bank, then the 1% of remaining calcium would be the vital currency in circulation that maintains the body's physiological economy. That whole economy is delicately controlled as we shall see shortly, not only by the central bank (the bone) but also by the National Mint (the diet) and by Foreign Exchange (the kidneys).

There are many other functions that calcium performs for each of us on a daily basis. It is critical to cardiac electrophysiology (helping to generate each heartbeat) and to the heart muscle's contractible strength (how much push the pump can deliver). Calcium also plays an essential role in the continuos control of blood pressure. (Hence, you can easily understand the widespread use of calcium – channel blockers as drugs for heart disease and hypertension). The process of blood clotting, so essential for protection from bleeding to death, is influenced directly by circulating calcium which activates clotting factors. Many enzyme systems utilize calcium as an important mineral cofactor, and several hormones either derive from the effects of calcium or exert their influence with calcium participation. Even the process of cell deletion or apoptosis (by fragmentation into membrane-bound particles which are engulfed or phagocytosed by other cells) involves calcium. In a single word, without calcium human life is impossible and we die.

Yet the body focuses on the small fraction of mobile calcium in the blood, for that is far more important for survival than the stored calcium in the bone. We survive not so much because of the tensile strength of our bones, but rather through the sophistication and specialization of deployed cells. That is why clinicians must measure blood serum calcium levels a thousand times more often than we do bone density. Life is compatible within only a narrow range of such "total serum calcium" levels. It's a critical parameter in the state of equilibrium in the body – otherwise called 'homeostasis.'

CALCIUM HOMEOSTATIS

The small fraction of body calcium that circulates in the blood exists as free ionized calcium (50%) or bound to proteins (40%) or to phosphate or citrate ligands. Nature values the fine control of the serum calcium levels so much, that there are three different cooperative mechanisms that regulate the level of this circulating mineral. They operate in the gut, the kidney and the bone.

Calcium is present in a wide range of foods as we shall see and when consumed it is absorbed from **the intestine**. It is transported into the body by a special carrier protein which requires vitamin D for its synthesis. Vitamin D itself is derived from dietary sources, plus the body manufactures its own vitamin D upon exposure to sunlight. Good sources of vitamin D include cod liver oil, cold water fish (such as mackerel, salmon, herring), butter and egg yolks. Today, severe vitamin D deficiency is rare in the developed world, but partly because it is not uncommon to have vitamin D added to calcium sources, as in fortified milk or calcium supplements. (More on that later).

A number of substances can inhibit the absorption of calcium. High protein present in the gut at the same time can bind to the calcium to reduce its absorption. Phytic acid, found in bran, whole cereals and raw vegetables will do the same thing. Uronic acid, a component of dietary fiber, and oxalic acid found in certain fruits and vegetables, can also bind calcium. However, diets habitually high in these acids are not thought to have a major effect on calcium absorption. Saturated fats can also reduce the net absorption of calcium.

One other factor influencing calcium absorption from the intestine is an endogenous hormone called parathyroid hormone (PTH). This hormone is secreted by a few small glands adjacent to the thyroid (hence, para-thyroid). In excess, it acts on the gut by increasing the production of the active metabolite of vitamin D to increase calcium absorption, and on the kidney to increase reabsorption of calcium in the tubules of the kidney.

That brings us to the second controlling mechanism for calcium homeostatis: **the kidney**. Calcium is excreted and reabsorbed in the kidney and the net retention is influenced directly by this parathyroid hormone. This process is totally by internal (endogenous) control, as nature dictates. Calcium is lost in the urine, faeces and sweat. In adults, calcium loss is made roughly equal to dietary calcium. If dietary calcium is low, calcium loss is reduced. Or, if calcium intake is increased too high, then more calcium is lost in turn. Adaptation to both high and low calcium intakes can therefore occur naturally. Reduced intake leads to increased efficiency of absorption and decreased renal excretion. In infants and growing children, calcium is retained for new bone growth. Calcium is also lost during lactation in breast milk and needs to be replaced.

When calcium intake is inadequate to replace obligatory total calcium losses, in order to maintain the necessary serum calcium levels, there is a change in normal **bone metabolism.** Bone is constantly being remodeled. Some constructive cells called *osteoblasts* are constantly active adding calcium to the structural bone matrix. Other destructive cells called *osteoclasts* dissolve bone and remove calcium from that storage to mobilize it into the bloodstream. They are the two types of bankers in the body's calcium economy: one deposits and one withdraws. The relative activity is again controlled by parathyroid hormone, by another (polypeptide) hormone called thyrocalcitonin, by active vitamin D and by local cell metabolites (especially in some cancers). When calcium is lost from the bone in order to maintain a balance of serum calcium as first priority, the bone density is reduced. Over time, the bones can become brittle and liable to fracture – a condition known as osteoporosis. More about this too, later.

The body utilizes all three of these mechanisms – the gut, the kidney and the bone – to keep the circulating calcium level where it should be. Most of the time, success is achieved. Otherwise, there are clinical consequences. When the level is too high (*hypercalcemia*), with an incidence of 4/1000/year of the population, it is a result of too much parathyroid hormone 90% of the time. In a hospital setting, it is a leading sign for malignant disease. Many would have no symptoms, but those who do (40-50%) might have any of the following: loss of appetite, nausea and vomiting, constipation, weakness and lethargy, lots of drinking and urinating, depression, stupor or psychosis. It is a treatable condition.

When the serum calcium level is too low (*hypocalcemia*) the most characteristic sign is a triad of muscle spasms, a noisy high-pitched respiration (stridor), and convulsions. This is often the result of kidney failure or of deficiency in vitamin D activity or parathyroid hormone. This is even more easily corrected, although it too could become a serious emergency if neglected or left unmanaged.

There are other intrinsic metabolic bone diseases related to calcium deficiency. In children, lack of vitamin D can lead to an inability to calcify the bone matrix – a condition known as **rickets**. This is uncommon today but it is associated with skeletal deformities, susceptibility to fractures, weakness and disturbances of growth. In adults, the similar condition can lead to **osteomalacia** which can be diagnosed by examining biopsy samples of bone under the microscope, to find general bone loss with widened osteoid seams in the uncalcified bone. The presentation of osteomalacia is not as dramatic as rickets, but the major symptoms include diffuse skeletal pain, bone tenderness, fractures, gait disturbance and muscle weakness. Both conditions are treatable.

By far the most prevalent bone disease related to calcium is the group of diseases with diverse causes but all labeled as osteoporosis (porous bone), where the reduction in the density of the bone is inadequate for mechanical support.

OSTEOPOROSIS

Osteoporosis is a major public health threat for more than 28 million Americans, 80 percent of whom are older women. In the US today, about 10 million individuals already have the disease and 18 million more have low bone mass, placing them at increased risk for osteoporosis. Significant risk has been reported in people of all ethnic backgrounds although the risk among African-Americans is noticeably lower. Yet as much as 85% of osteoporosis sufferers in America go untreated. It is a disease vastly underdiagnosed.

This disease can be devastating in its consequences, especially in the elderly. The incidence increases with age and 50% of all people over 75, both men and women, will be affected by the disease. It is responsible for 1.3-1.5 million fractures each year mainly in the hip, vertebrae and wrist, and these place a burden worth more than $15 billion /year ($40 million plus every day) on the healthcare system. More women die from osteoporosis in the U.S. than from breast cancer, uterine cancer and cervical cancer *combined*. Osteoporosis is the #3 uncured disease, behind only heart disease and arthritis. Vertebral crush fractures or traumatic hip fractures can instantly reduce the life expectancy of a formerly robust senior citizen from decades to a few months. Crush fractures may occur spontaneously during daily activities such as coughing, lifting, bending, arising from a sitting chair, or even from an enthusiastic hug. Often these crush fractures occur within the vertebrae (vertebra crush fractures) and can cause severe pain, "dowagers hump" (stooped over, with bulging back) and significant loss of height (up to even 5-8 inches). Hip fractures can cripple permanently. It is not uncommon for seniors to arrive at the emergency room with a hip fracture, not because they fell, but rather because they had a fracture that caused them to fall, sometimes with secondary complications. In 75% of the cases, the vertebral fractures are insidiously "silent". But once a fracture occurs, the patient typically has a 1 in 5 chance of re-fracturing within the next year. Multiple fractures markedly reduce life expectancy. As many as 50% of all patients on oral steroid therapy will suffer an osteoporosis – induced fracture, and 17% within the first year of therapy.

We already hinted that certain people are more likely to develop osteoporosis than others. The list of risk factors for this disease include all of the following:

- Being female
- Thin and/or small frame
- Advanced age
- A family history of osteoporosis (1st degree relative)
- Post-menopause, including both early (premature ovarian failure) or surgically-induced menopause
- Abnormal absence of menstrual periods (amenorrhea)
- Anorexia nervosa or bulimia
- A diet low in calcium, vitamin D/low sun exposure
- Use of certain medications, such as corticosteroids and anticonvulsants
- Low testosterone levels in men

- An inactive lifestyle (low weight-bearing exercise)
- Cigarette smoking
- Excessive use of alcohol
- Being Asian or Caucasian (especially Scandinavian)

Several of the risk factors just listed should suggest appropriate changes in lifestyle for those at risk. Although there are some treatments of limited benefit after a fracture is experienced or the silent disease is diagnosed, the obvious focus in osteoporosis must be on prevention. The goal is to build strong, dense bones, especially earlier in life. A key strategy to help prevent osteoporosis is to have an adequate intake of calcium preferably starting from early childhood but certainly before age 30. Actually, by about age 20, the average woman has acquired 98% of her skeletal mass so building strong bones during childhood and adolescence can be the best defense against developing osteoporosis later.

A recent article in the *American Journal of Clinical Nutrition* sought to review the answer to the question 'Can early milk calcium consumption strengthen bones later in life?' The answer is YES! They showed that previous milk consumption was associated with greater bone density in young women. The results were consistent with the hypothesis that higher milk intake during adolescence, is associated with greater total body, spine and radial bone mineral measured during the development of peak bone mass (approximately age 30), whereas current calcium intakes may influence spine bone mineral content. In addition, milk intake at a younger age, may contribute to similar habits of milk intake later in life. The bottom line is that it makes good sense to encourage young people (especially young girls) to get copious amounts of calcium in their youth.

There are a few other illnesses that are now frequently attributed to calcium for one reason or another. Perhaps, the most obvious one is the relationship to kidney stones.

KIDNEY STONES

If osteoporosis is the associated consequence with insufficient calcium intake, then the opposite result from too much dietary calcium might be presumed to be kidney stones. But again, we must not rush to judgement.

Kidney stones (renal calculi, to be more precise) are common and generally preventable. They are of different types or composition with calcium oxalate or mixed calcium oxalate and phosphate comprising as much as 80% of the total. Most of the others are struvite or infected stones with triple phosphate (calcium, magnesium and ammonium phosphate), and uric acid stones. Altogether they are more common in young adults and tend to recur in the same individual. The stones are crystalline precipitates formed in the urine as it is filtered out in the renal system. There are a combination of risk factors which (essentially) combine the tendency to excessive supersaturation of the urine and/or low inhibition of crystal formation. The key physiological observation to point out is that at least 95% of patients with calcium stones have normal *serum* calcium levels. Yet about 60-70% of these same patients have elevated calcium in their urine. Some 25-40% form calcium stones with even normal calcium levels in their *urine*. Problems can arise when there are either imbalances in the controlling hormones (especially PTH); or abnormalities in kidney function; or insufficient urine volume, or excessive bone resorption. Therefore, it is incorrect to make a direct connection between calcium intake in normal individuals and the formation of kidney stones.

It is indeed possible to even go a step further. Dietary calcium intake has been shown to be *inversely* associated with the major calcium oxalate kidney stone formation. In a recent article in *European Urology*, animal fat intake but not dietary calcium intake was associated with stone formation. In a British prospective study of non-medical prophylaxis after a first kidney stone, almost 80% of 242 patients reported a high intake of meat and a low intake of dairy products. Among a cohort of 27,001 Finnish male smokers aged 50-69 years who were initially free of kidney stones, calcium intake was not associated with the risk of stones. For further reading on this issue, the reader should note that the role of calcium in the *prevention* of kidney stones was also just recently reviewed.

Thus, since there are internal regulation mechanisms in the gut, kidney and bone, and the important serum calcium levels is strictly controlled in normal individuals, one need not become too anxious about overloading on dietary calcium if kidney function is essentially normal. The opposite is not true, since inadequate calcium intake which does not replace the natural losses, will lead to increased bone resorption and the potential pathological consequences.

The question arises then, how much calcium should a normal individual ingest on a daily basis?

CALCIUM INTAKE

The daily amount of calcium needed is defined in several different ways.

In the United States:
- Recommended Dietary Allowances (RDAs) are the amount of vitamins and minerals needed to provide for adequate nutrition in most healthy persons. RDAs for a given nutrient may vary depending on a person's age, sex, and physical condition (e.g. pregnancy).
- Daily Values (DVs) are used on food and dietary supplement labels to indicate the percent of the recommended daily amount of each nutrient that a serving provides. DV replaces the previous designation of United States Recommended Daily Allowances (USRDAs)

In Canada:
- Recommended Nutrient Intakes (RNIs) are used to determine the amounts of vitamins, minerals and protein needed to provide adequate nutrition and lessen the risk of chronic disease.

The normal daily recommended intakes for calcium among various age groups in the U.S. and Canada are summarized in Table 10.

Getting the proper amount of calcium in the diet every day and participating in weight-bearing exercise (walking, dancing, bicycling, aerobics, jogging), especially during the early years of life (up to about 35 years of age) is most important in helping to build and maintain

Table 10.	Normal daily recommended intakes for calcium (mg)	
Person	U.S. (mg)	Canada (mg)
Infants and children		
Birth to 3 years of age	400-800	250-550
4 to 6 years of age	800	600
7 to 10 years of age	800	700-1100
Adolescent and adult males	800-1200	800-1100
Adolescent and adult females	800-1200	700-1100
Pregnant females	1200	1200-1500
Breast-feeding females	1200	1200-1500

bones as dense as possible to prevent the development of osteoporosis in later life.

During pregnancy, calcium absorption from the gut increases and no additional calcium is generally needed although it is generally prudent to supplement the normal diet. Pregnant adolescents in particular are the exception to this, having especially high calcium needs. Breast feeding women need an extra 550 mg of calcium daily to replace their losses which can be as high as 300 mg or more in daily breast milk. The elderly should also be aware since calcium absorption decreases with age.

Can we get adequate calcium from our diets?

Yes, we can, in principle. However, as we age, we absorb less calcium and vitamin D, and manufacture less vitamin D in the skin following skin exposure. Just think that we absorb in reality, only about 10% of the calcium we eat. You would have to drink about one quart of milk daily to get your recommended *minimum* intake of calcium. Most adults (and children too) simply do not do this. The U.S. National Institutes for Health (NIH) believe that the vast majority of Americans have an inadequate intake of calcium (despite the intensive dairy advertising). A recent NIH consensus committee of experts found that the current RDA for calcium was too low for older adults.

A short list of some calcium rich foods is shown in Table 11. Note the copious calcium content in some non-dairy foods like tofu, figs, salmon or collard greens. Some foods interfere with calcium absorption and should be avoided. A brief list is shown in Table 12. Calcium from fruits and vegetables is in an unchelated, elemental form and not very easily absorbed. Additionally, phytates and oxylates found in green leafy vegetables such as spinach, bind to calcium, making it less available for absorption. Oxylates found in some plants, could be problematic for persons prone to oxylate kidney stone formation.

When all is said and done, there is still a good rationale for calcium supplementation.

CALCIUM SUPPLEMENTATION

Dietary surveys have repeatedly shown inadequate intake of calcium in North America. Many health authorities recommend that both teenagers and the elderly consume 1500 mg of calcium a day and translate that into four to five servings of milk or dairy foods. It is also recommended that children and adults under 50 years of age get 1000 mg or three to four servings from the dairy group. But even so, less than 5-10% of Americans meet those targets. The fact that leafy green vegetables, fortified orange juice and some soy foods like tofu are also good sources hardly makes a change because food choices in North America are skewed in the wrong direction.

The ideal obviously would be to get adequate calcium on a daily basis from the regular foods we eat. However, those who consume a diet with insufficient calcium (and that may include most people in North America) could use calcium supplements to make up the difference. There are a wide variety of calcium supplements on the market today and most physicians will readily prescribe calcium supplements for their patients. The major indications for medical calcium supplementation are osteoporosis (porous bone), osteopenia (weakened or diminished bones) and during pregnancy and lactation. Calcium is one of the very few nutritional supplements for which the US Food and Drug Administration will allow medical claims.

Calcium-Rich Foods
Table 11.   Calcium Content of Selected Foods

Food	Serving Size	Calcium Content (mg)
Parmesan cheese, grated	1 ounce	390
Collards, cooked from frozen	½ cup	179
Sardines, canned in oil	2 sardines	92
Kale, boiled	½ cup	47
Yogurt (lowfat, fruit-flavored)	8 ounces	314
Gruyere cheese	1 ounce	287
Milk, skim	1 cup	302
Blackstrap molasses	1 tablespoon	172
Figs, dried	10 figs	269
Cheddar cheese (American)	1 ounce	211
Creamed cottage cheese	1 cup	126
Broccoli, boiled	½ cup	36
American, cheese, processed	1 ounce	124
Salmon, canned (pink)	3 ounces	181
Tofu, raw, firm	½ cup	258
Calcium-fortified orange juice	6 ounces	200
Calcium-fortified cereals	1 cup	300

• From JAT Pennington and HN Church, *Bowes and Church's Food Values of Portions Commonly Used.* 16th ed, Philadelphia: JB Lippincott, 1994

Table 12.
FOODS TO AVOID FOR EFFICIENT
CALCIUM APSORPTION

Carbonated cola drinks
Legumes and wheat bran
High fat foods and foods high in saturated fats
Large amounts of chocolate
Excessive alcohol
Excessive coffee
Aspartame sweetener and excessive sugar
Heavily chlorinated or fluoridated tap water
Caffeine
Salt
Animal protein

From more recent research, it seems that there is even more benefit to be derived from regular calcium intake than just the strength of bones and teeth. In the famous Nurses Health Study, after 14 years of follow-up of some 85,764 U.S. women, researchers just reported last year, their findings that women who had "the largest calcium intake had 31% lower adjusted relative risk of ischemic stroke. Other researchers investigating the potential roles of calcium and vitamin D in colon and breast cancer prevention, reported also last year that many cases of colon cancer may be prevented with regular intake of calcium in the range of 1800 mg per day. A published review of 27 studies looking at the association of milk and colorectal cancer discovered an impressive amount of evidence for milk's protective, anti-cancer effects. Calcium is believed to bind excess fat and bile in the gut, causing potentially toxic compounds to precipitate and pass out of the body. Other studies suggest that calcium helps keep cell growth of the colon lining in check. Rapid and abnormal cell proliferation is an early warning sign of possible cancerous growth. Much more research is needed in this area.

An interesting double-blind study on the effect of calcium in relieving symptoms of PMS (premenstrual syndrome) may be of special interest to women. Dr. Thys-Jacobs discovered that compared to the women without PMS, women with PMS have abnormally low levels of calcium at the time of ovulation. She and other researchers at St. Luke's-Roosevelt Hospital Center in New York then looked at the effect in nearly 500 women affected by PMS and comprising a cross-section of the population. The results provided strong evidence that calcium supplements can effectively treat a wide variety of PMS symptoms. The effect was more pronounced with successive cycles over the few cycles that these women were studied.

So, for more than one reason, it would appear that calcium supplementation does make good sense. All the natural calcium supplements have the calcium attached to different organic groups such as carbonate, phosphate, citrate etc., in the form of calcium salts. The question then is, does the source or form of calcium as a supplement really matter? The answer is again an unequivocal YES!

The most common source of calcium as a supplement is calcium carbonate (for example, Os-Cal™ or Caltrate™). This is essentially 'food grade' chalk. It contains 40% elemental calcium (500 mg $CaCO_3$ = 20 mg Ca) in an inorganic salt that comes as tablets including chewable tablets (usually flavored), and as capsules or oral suspensions. Calcium carbonate reacts with the acid in the stomach to form a more ionized, inorganic form of calcium which can then be absorbed. It is an effective antacid and is marketed as such (like Tums™ or Maalox™) with copious calcium as a useful ingredient. The quality of calcium carbonate tablets varies widely. Some break up and dissolve far too slowly in the stomach to be effectively absorbed. A simple home-test would be to try dissolving the tablets in warm water or white vinegar, with occasional stirring, for up to 30 minutes. If it has not dissolved, consider it unlikely to be absorbed by the body. Chewable and liquid calcium supplements dissolve much better.

The second most common form of calcium as a supplement is calcium citrate (like Citrical™). It contains only 21% elemental calcium (500 mg = 100 mg Ca), but it is better absorbed than calcium carbonate and can be taken on an empty stomach since it is less dependent on stomach acid. The downside is that it requires twice as much to get the same amount of elemental calcium. Then there is calcium lactate which is the third most common form. It contains only 13% elemental calcium by weight (500 mg = 65 mg Ca). This is relatively well absorbed in low-stomach acid states but again, much larger quantities must be used due to the low calcium content. Perhaps the best absorbed and tolerated of all the calcium compounds is the more organic calcium gluconate. It is a relatively rare form containing only a mere 9% of calcium by weight (500 mg = 45 mg Ca). In this case, one must take 4-5 times as much as calcium carbonate.

With the high demand for calcium supplements, the market has been flooded by calcium products that have not always met the best criteria based on the individual's needs for purity, absorbability, tolerance, convenience, cost and availability in selecting any calcium supplement for safety and efficacy.

PURE MILK CALCIUM

When the public thinks of dietary calcium, thanks to all the advertising and promotion by the dairy industry and its lobby, it thinks more often than not of milk. No wonder, dairy foods provide 75% of the calcium in the U.S. diet. And why not? After all, milk is an excellent source of calcium and calcium from milk is one of the most (if not the most) bioavailable forms of calcium. But as we have seen earlier in this book (see Chapter Two), many people have reservations about the high, regular consumption of milk for a variety of reasons: the fat content, lactose intolerance, potential contamination, the consequences of pasteurization and homogenization, and more. We also pointed out that drinking milk was not a simple and straightforward issue for maintaining bone calcium. Otherwise, we would observe a one-to-one correspondence between milk consumption and bone health, for example. The major problem of osteoporosis is more prevalent in the developed world where milk consumption is relatively common. Even within that population, the evidence that drinking milk per se is the answer, is neither complete nor compelling.

Now, thanks to the application of modern technology, it is possible to get all the benefits of pure milk calcium without any of the downsides of whole milk consumption. Using a proprietary extraction technology continued with further purification techniques, scientists have been able to isolate the rich calcium from milk, with no fat, lactose, cholesterol, hormones, antibiotics or any environmental contaminants that cause so many consumers to have apprehension about drinking a lot of milk. The Pure Milk Calcium™ so derived contains 24% of elemental and highly absorbable calcium by weight (500 mg = 120 mg Ca). It is highly soluble and digestible and supplied in tablets containing 250 mg of elemental calcium and 100 IU of vitamin D. It is real calcium from pure milk, another gem from nature's goldmine. In general, calcium is most effective when taken in small amounts throughout the day and Pure Milk Calcium may be taken any time during the day with or without meals.

This form of calcium supplementation with the calcium from whey mineral complex (WMC) has been shown to result in superior bone density and resistance to breaking, in growing animals fed WMC compared to animals fed calcium carbonate or calcium from powdered bone. Pure Milk Calcium builds greater (8% more) bone density than calcium carbonate. The bones developed show 7% higher levels of calcium. This unique product also contains 13% phosphorus to give a calcium/phosphorus ratio similar to the human body.

SHOULD I USE A CALCIUM SUPPLEMENT

Experts agree that individuals should get as much of their recommended daily intake of calcium from food sources. If that's impossible, a calcium-rich diet, combined with a calcium supplement can be a good compromise.

1. Assess your risk of getting osteoporosis: youth, females, family history, post menopause, seniors, smokers, inactivity etc.
2. Review your diet for adequate calcium sources.
3. Choose a supplement with the ideal combination of calcium and vitamin D. Although it is popular to add magnesium to a calcium supplement, this is not recommended, because of the not infrequent and unpleasant side effects.
4. Limit the amount of calcium per supplement dosage to 500 mg, since many foods are supplemented with calcium. In fact, the aver-

age American obtains 500-600 mg/day of calcium from their diet. There is no benefit to exceeding 2,000 mg of calcium per day.

5. Look for a supplement with a low recommended dosage that is taken several times a day. Calcium is best absorbed by the body in small amounts.

6. Increase supplement intake gradually. Take 250 mg to 500 mg a day for a week, then add more calcium slowly.

7. Choose a supplement that can be taken at any time of day, and not specifically with meals. It is important to note that calcium carbonate combinations must be taken with meals since they can be hard on the stomach.

8. Avoid calcium from unrefined oyster shell, bone meal or dolomite. The FDA has issued warnings that bone meal and dolomite could be dangerous because these products may contain lead or other heavy metals.

9. Ensure your supplement is easily absorbed by the body, is well tolerated and contains an adequate fraction of elemental calcium.

10. Drink lots of fluid with your calcium supplement.

But what is pure milk anyway? This gold mine from nature derives from the modern dairy farm. In the next chapter, we go on a personal visit. Please join us now.

Chapter Eleven

A VISIT TO A MODERN DAIRY FARM

Life in the city is a riot. The noise of automobiles and traffic congestion; the imposing claustrophobia of tall, concrete and glass buildings, rising above the narrow streets; the tide of human bodies hustling past, waxing and waning through the rush hour; the smell of polluted air –whoever designed to live there? But over the past century, by the millions we came. To Mexico City, with its large, sprawling urban ghettoes; to New York City, a city that never sleeps, where stress and fear are normalized but never neutralized; to Quebec City, where power converged as governments sat and sometimes democracy ruled – and to all the cities, large and small – where nature gives way to commerce, and where green becomes gray, neon lights block out the sunset, and air becomes smog; where sounds of animals and birds are substituted by loud sirens and horns. Whatever became of stillness and silence!

Out there somewhere, is another reality. A place we call the country. There is still such a place, where the grass grows and the cows graze and the birds sing. It is a rural tranquility, with still waters and flowing streams; where the trees still provide shade, when there's no one else to hide. Through all the changing scenes and seasons, life goes on, without the city and all it has to offer – but not vice versa. From here, the farmer feeds the city, the nation and the world.

Let's go for a visit. Let's go find out what really happens behind the scenes to allow urban dwellers like me (and possibly like you, too) to go to the local supermarket at any time and find fresh food and produce, including the staple milk and dairy products.

We must leave the city but we do not quite leave it behind, for soon we discover that even on a modern dairy farm, there is the impact of the computer revolution; the application of modern genetics and biotechnology; the sophistication of the latest techniques in refrigeration and transportation. What has really happened over the past one hundred years is that we have changed from what essentially was an agricultural food supply, to an industrial food supply. The old family farm, where one generation taught the next to sit on stools and milk cows by hand – that's almost completely a thing of the past. Urbanization and high density living, demanded that food be available in large quantities, since fewer and fewer farmers would have to feed more and more mouths. Only centralization could afford the economy of scale and rationalize the distribution of farm products across over-crowded cities. Survival became economics.

And so our visit today will not take us to a homestead where the farmer and his family have a few dozen cows grazing in the fields and milk just enough to distribute in the surrounding communities. Rather, it is part of a vast network of factory farms (or farming factories, which might be a better term, since the emphasis is now on production) that produces a product quota, to rigorous standard specifications, on a tight production schedule. The traditional family farm has been transformed into (or replaced by) a modern dairy (factory) farm.

The one we visit today is 40 miles outside the city and it is a relatively small dairy farm in the northeast. It has a capacity of 330 registered Holstein dairy cattle, including 160 mature cows and 170 replacement heifers and young calves. The milking herd is kept in a unique combination of a 128 tie-stall barn and a 48-unit free-stall barn which have common access to a 16-unit double-eight herring bone parlor. Maternity and physiology wings are also serviced with milking equipment for the cows kept in these areas. There are three nurseries located alongside the maternity area for pre-weaned calves, plus a group housing heifer barn and a transition area for freshening heifers entering the milking herd. The entire operation is on less than 10 acres.

This is a relatively small dairy farm. Many North American farms have numbers of cows in the thousands, rather than hundreds, but the size of our farm today is not that uncommon. In the State of Colorado for example, there are 84,000 dairy cows living on 221 dairy farms, averaging 380 per farm, just 15% more than the farm we are visiting today. There is an economy of scale as the size of the farm increases, but then there is the increased capital cost and complex attendant problems of management, operations and maintenance.

RESEARCH

As we approach the farm today, it is obvious that this is not the traditional grazing pasture with the cows in the field and the farmer in the dell. There's no more waiting here 'til the cows come home. In fact, but for the sign at the entrance gate, one could hardly know what was going on inside the industrial-style buildings which back on to open but empty fields. The sign suggests that this is more than just a farm. It is a cutting-edge establishment, affiliated to a nearby rural university. Here the associated faculty and staff conduct research in genetics, nutrition, physiology, health, welfare, management and the environment. Among the areas of special interest, **reproduction research** has focused on the evaluation of a highly interventionist approach for managing reproduction in postpartum dairy cattle. This study will investigate the effect of an additive contribution of a number of reproduction therapies on reproductive efficiency.

Two **udder health trials** are underway on this farm. The first study is investigating the efficiency of a teat barrier formulation for reducing the incidence of intramammary infection during the dry period. The second study involves the evaluation of one diagnostic kit's ability to provide etiological information in a timely fashion, which will hopefully aid in the rational and targeted use of antibiotics by dairy producers.

Behavioral research here involves the study of dairy cows involved in the Automatic Milk System (AMS). These cows are being studied and compared against a control group to determine whether latent learning techniques could enhance or simplify the training process when dairy cows are just introduced to the AMS. This study is also comparing milk yields and manifestation of estrus signs (in heat) of these dairy cows.

This type of research work on a dairy farm is not common, but it is a reminder as we enter the gates that this is modern technology at work. Every aspect and phase of the dairy farm system that we are about to witness and describe has been studied by the scientific method. It is the product of many decades of rigorous and unbiased research driven by a desire to improve efficiency and productivity as well as animal welfare and ecological balance.

As we enter the first building we go down a corridor past the management offices where desktop computers process and store information on almost every aspect of the entire operation. At the click of a mouse, any cow in residence can be brought on to a computer screen and every detail of its existence can be displayed. It has a registered identification in a national database which points to its pedigree, its birth characteristics and every significant event in its life thereafter: its nutrition history, its milking history (every single milking is recorded in time, duration and quantity), its complete medical history, and much, much more.

HOUSING

Since our focus today is on the animals, let's pass the offices and computers and go directly to them where they spend the vast majority of their time. They live most of their lives in cow houses, rather than in the open fields. On our farm today, as we mentioned earlier, the larger barn for the milking cows is of the tie-stall variety which has 128 spaces, and the smaller barn which is a 48-unit free-stall barn. The younger hiefers are housed separately as a group in a different barn, and then there is the transition area.

The first stop in our visit is in the tie-stall Barn. As we open the door and step inside, there is no doubt remaining as to where exactly we are. The sights, the sounds, the smells … all tell the same story. This is indeed a dairy farm.

Smaller dairy herds are usually housed in a **tie-stall barn**. The name refers to how the cows are held in place in their stalls. A strap and a chain that hold the cow are attached to a bar in front of each cow's head. Each stall has just about one-and-a-half times the floor space that the cow occupies giving some room for movement but obviously limiting the same. The cow is free to stand, to lie, to go about a foot or so, back and forth, and not very much more. Each one gets a period of daily exercise when they are taken outside, again in groups, to a half acre paddock equipped with water stations where they are free to walk around as much as they choose. In addition, they make two scheduled trips to the milking parlor every day. Each time they leave their stalls, the strap and chain are easily released.

Confinement to these stalls has been a subject of much controversy. Agribusiness companies are quick to point out that animals in such 'factory farms' are "as well cared for as their own pets at home". Their basic needs are generously provided for. They are spared all the hazards and challenges that they might experience in the wild. They are nursed and attended with professional care. Yes, they do become the apple of someone's eye, a treasure to be preserved. But that may be an exaggeration. Other special interests such as the Humane Farming Association (HFA) insist that the basic needs of exercise and fresh air are inadequately addressed. These animals live an unnatural existence, with little or no autonomy. They exist only to serve the needs of others in the biosphere. Their style is cramped, their immunity compromised and their pleasure curtailed. One veterinarian observes that "when animals are intensively confined and under stress, as they are on factory farms, their autoimmune systems are affected and they are prone to infection and much more."

Here on this farm today, the cows appear healthy, cooperative and well adjusted. Wise dairy farmers know that cows that are comfortable in their environment are healthier animals. Healthier animals have less stress and are higher *producers*. Stressed cows do not eat and drink as much as they otherwise might and so they do not reach their full potential. In the natural environment, a cow is designed to eat, lie down, eat, lie down, over and over again. Any housing system that makes it uncomfortable for her to lie down disrupts the natural cycle. Cows forced to stand for prolonged periods have reduced dry intake and lower milk production. They may also suffer from laminitis (foot inflammation), reduced longevity, weight loss and reproduction problems. A typical cow should spend half the time lying down (comfortably). They should also get up without striking the stall dividers and neck rail.

Many innovations have been introduced to make the stalls more comfortable. Research has shown that given the choice, cows preferred rubber mats over concrete, and rubber crumb-filled mattresses over the rubber mats. But rubber mats resulted in a greater incidence of swollen locks. Clean, clay-free sand, while somewhat hard on the manure disposal equipment, is one of the most economical and effective surfaces preferred by cows. Sand moves readily under a cow's stress points and forms to the shape of her body. Growth of mastitis-causing organisms is minimal and any sand spilled into the alley provides additional traction for the animals. On the floor surface of the stall is a natural padding of loose straw bedding which proves very comfortable for the animals. It is changed regularly to ensure cleanliness and good sanitation.

This barn today is naturally ventilated to afford air exchange that carriers away hot air and moisture. Poor ventilation would also result in heat stress and as much as 25 percent reduction in milk production. Because of the natural body heat, no additional heating is required even during winter.

In the tie-stall barn, each cow has its own feeding station immediately at the front of the stall and there is no fighting for feed space. All cows have free access to drinking water on demand. Each cow can eat over 100lbs (50kg) of food, and drink between 25-50 gallons (100 litres) of water each day. Their diet is balanced for energy, protein and forage. At the rear end of each row of stalls is a depressed trough to collect manure and urine, which is all moved along mechanically to a pit at the back of the barn and used elsewhere for fertilizer. (Often dairy cows are fed leftover products from manufacturing of food for humans. They help recycling by eating waste products produced in making cereals, cookies and other foods. It's all one eco-system.)

On this farm we are visiting, there is a small **free-stall Barn** of 48-units. Large dairy herds are typically housed in free-stall barns where it is easier to handle a larger number of cows and the farmer's work is not as heavy. In one part of this barn is the eating and sleeping area. Traffic flow permits a circular pattern to allow all animals access to waterers and to the feed bunk. Timid cows or younger heifers may be reluctant to enter a dead-end stall for fear of being trapped by a dominant herd-mate. Feed and water intake are encouraged with a 12-foot wide crossover for every 80 feet of alley to permit traffic flow past the waterers. By design, waterers in the crossovers offer a minimum of 21 feet of trough for every 100 cows. Down the middle of this whole area, tractors drive through to deposit the cows' food in the feed alleys.

Free stall barns have floor surfaces that provide cows with adequate traction. Every day a cow in free-stall housing can walk from 80 to 2500 meters (more than a mile). High stocking density or slippery floors will discourage movement, especially to subordinate cows. This would result in competition for restricted amounts of feed or limited bunk space. A properly prepared hexagonally-grooved floor is far superior to a smooth surface, which increases the risk of injury. The floors are cleaned frequently to avoid wet slippery surfaces.

Another type of shelter that is used by some farmers, especially where the weather is mild, is **loose housing**. Here the cows are allowed to move freely about in a sheltered area. All the cows have their budding horns cauterized in the first few weeks after birth to stunt their growth, so there are no available weapons for territorial fights at any time. These docile, productive animals just cooperate with the program.

FEEDING

On this particular farm, where most of the cows are housed in a tie-stall barn, the cows feed and drink freely on demand, just as they would if they were grazing in the open fields. Each cow's intake is carefully monitored every day, for that in itself is a symptom of good health or else of stress or disease in the animal. Needless to say, countless studies have been done to correlate dietary intake with milk production and animal health and longevity. All modern farms have optimized the food supply, especially since this could have a major impact on the economics of the operation. In one year a cow eats literally tons of food. Yet they have very little body fat because most of their food energy intake is used to produce milk. A typical cow on an average day might consume the following variety of foods:

- 8 – 10lb of hay
- 30-40lb of silage
- 20-25lb of mixed grains
- salt, vitamins and minerals
- 25-50 gallons of water

Silage is a mixture of grasses and grains that have been allowed to ferment in a silo. Together this amounts to about 75,000 kilocaries each day. Compare this to the typical person who eats about 2,000 kilocalories per day.

When a cow eats, she partially chews and then quickly swallows her food. This food goes into the first section of her stomach which actually has four compartments, each section of which has a different function. Food enters the large *rumen* which is only partially separated from the second compartment called the *reticulum*. These two essentially soften the food and hold it there until the cow is finished eating. The food forms into lumps the size of tennis balls, each called a cud. The cow then does something very different. She regurgitates the cuds into the mouth individually and then does a more thorough chewing. The re-chewed food is swallowed again, this time into the third compartment or *omasum* where softening and grinding of the food continues. Finally, the food reaches the fourth compartment, the *abomasum* where it is digested further. The small intestine completes the digestive process and the nutrients are then absorbed.

The cow's net intake and therefore the quality of her milk supply is determined by the quality of her food supply. This is rigorously controlled and monitored and even in modern dairy farming, with all the elaborate sophistication, feed additives are at a minimum and almost non-existent.

On other farms, where the cows are housed in free stalls, it is very important to have a good feeding-management system to promote intense feeding activity and normal social behavior. Cows cycle through the barn at least twice per day for milking and they must contend with periodic interruptions like herd health checks and manure management. There is constant grouping and regrouping according to age, lactation or production levels. All this plays upon the cow's natural need for social hierarchies.

As soon as the social order is established, feeding becomes the dominate drive. There are several highly competitive times at the feed bunk, particularly when fresh food is offered and when cows return from milking. On-farm research in western New York indicated a spike in feeding activity when feed is pushed up in front of cows, when fresh feed becomes available or after milking as cows are on their way back from the free stalls. The key is therefore to have plenty of feed available and ample bunk space to minimize the effect of competition. Irregular feeding intervals, overcrowding, excessive walking required to and from the parlor, or insufficient bunk space, are all impediments to feeding behavior.

There's also a long running argument in the dairy industry about whether grazing or conventional confinement systems are more profitable. A recent grazing study at the University of Wisconsin showed that average returns from management-intensive rotational grazing (MIRG) compares more than favorably with those from conventional dairying in the State of Wisconsin. MIRG lets cows harvest a significant amount of the forage for themselves. That's the major difference. It can be done with or without other practices and technologies such as seasonal calving, milking parlors, total mixed rations and so on. In Wisconsin, grazing is an increasingly popular practice, up to 23 percent of dairy farms in 1999. Cows on nearly half of Wisconsin's dairy farms grazed pastures to meet some of their forage needs in 1999.

But the farm we are visiting today is not in Wisconsin. It is one belonging to the more common and conventional confinement system. Everything is programmed here for maximum efficiency and the clock rules. So on cue ... the cows are untied (in groups of 16 at a time on this farm) ... the strap and chain are released ... and off they go ... its *milking time*!

MILKING

The cows follow the routine easily and conveniently. They file out of the barn, through the open gates and into the milking parlor nearby. When the cows come into the milking parlor they line up to stand in angled milking stalls. They seem so docile, so resigned and contented with their role. In this parlor today we get to observe them through the glass window of the spectator gallery. We have front row posts but we'd rather they not see us pressing our faces against the glass. They're in business and are not wishing to be distracted by our social niceties or salutations.

There are eight stalls on either side of this parlor to permit milking 16 cows at one time by a single farmer. On larger dairy farms, the milking parlor might accommodate up to 40 or 50 cows at a time. Between the two rows of these cow stalls is a pit where the farmer stands to attack the milking equipment. This is so much easier because the farmer does not have to bend down to the cow's level to milk her. Each cow is carefully identified. She wears a numbered neck bracelet for visual recognition and carries an electronic transponder which feeds directly into the computer. There are stainless steel pipes with shut off valves and computerized liquid-crystal displays, everywhere. The whole operation looks sophisticated and in some sense it is.

Hopefully, since it's milking time, each cow's udder is now full of milk. The udder is a large pouch on the underside of the cow, with four compartments inside. Each compartment has a teat for the milk to be sucked out. The milking machine has four corresponding cups, one for each teat. These cups pump the milk gently and rhythmically from the cow's udder. Before the rubber suction cups are fitted on to the cow's teats, the farmer washes her teats with a disinfectant solution, then he/she carefully rinses and dries them. This is good practice but certainly not universal. A major 1997 survey of thousands of dairy farmers in Ontario revealed their milking habits. Sixty five percent of survey respondents used a wet wash and dry udder preparation *before* milking. Close to 30 percent used a pre-milking teat disinfectant, compared to almost 60 percent in the US. This may reflect the larger herd size since U.S. data suggest that the larger the herd, the more likely it is to use a pre-milking teat dip. Strangely enough, the Ontario farmers were more rigorous about post-milking care than their U.S. neighbors. As many as 94 percent of the same survey respondents said they performed teat disinfection *after* milking, while the U.S. figure stands only at 80 percent. The survey also found that teat dipping is more popular than spraying, in Ontario at least. Udder health is critical to the entire operation. Herds that practice improper udder preparation before milking have a five times greater chance of having *Staph. aureus* bacteria cultured from their cows.

The action of the milking machine imitates that of milking by hand and takes less than five minutes for each cow. Milking the cows by hand or by machine never really hurts the cow. Here on this farm today, just as was done for hundreds of years, the cow is milked regularly early in the morning and late in the afternoon. Milking times vary from farm to farm, and some milk three times a day rather than two. This milking routine happens on the farm everyday of every week of every year. Every detail for each and every cow is computerized.

After each group of sixteen has been milked, the machines are removed, the gates open on the other end of the parlor, and they leave, contented and relieved, to mend their way slowly back to the barn for more of the same. Day in and day out - they eat, they lie, they sleep, they eat, they milk, they eat some more. Once a day, they get their brief time of exercising, walking outside in the haddock. Then it's back inside again for more of the same routines. It's a cow's life!

The milk obtained directly from the cows is weighed and then carried by stainless steel pipes from the milking machines to a large refrigerated bulk tank across the hall from the milking parlor. En route it passes through a pre-cooler which drops the temperature by up to 20°C before it goes into the computer-controlled refrigerated tank. On some farms they may even use well water of about 12°C to pre-cool the milk and then the tempered water is then given to the cows. One can feel the difference in temperature between the input and output pipes. The milk is coming out of the pre-cooler so cold in fact, that the cooler itself only runs typically for half an hour after milking. By the third or fourth milking in the tank, the temperature never goes above 4°C. The milk from the cow is in the tank at this temperature within 90 seconds from leaving the cow. The faster it cools down the better.

Every second day the milk is piped from the bulk tank (which on this farm has a 12,000 litre capacity) into a tank truck which visits the farm. The truck makes regular calls at farms on its route following a very strict schedule to ensure rapid transfer of milk to the plant. Each truck driver is a licensed milk grader. He takes samples of milk into sterilized bottles which are stored in the truck for delivery to the testing laboratory. He hauls the milk to the dairy where it is tested routinely for a number of important quality control variables: bacterial counts, parasites, antibiotics, somatic cell counts, milk fat content etc. All this data is again computerized and provides a very efficient tracking system. Any milk delivery batch that fails to meet rigorous quality control standards are rejected at the dairy and fines are often imposed as a penalty in order to keep the systems operational and the farmers honest.

After each cycle, the whole system is washed with detergent, acid rinse and chlorine rinse.

Recommended Milking Procedures

The quality of milk obtained from the cow is crucial in maintaining high dairy standards. Each farm has its own standardized routines which, when appropriately followed, yields a highly quality product to send to the dairy every single time. Just for completeness, here are some key instructions for the milker on the farm we are visiting today:

- **Provide a clean, low stress environment for cows.**

    Cows that are frightened or excited before milking may not have a normal milk letdown response in spite of an effective preparation routine. Stress hormones increase the risk of mastitis.
- **Check foremilk and udder for mastitis.**

    Physical examination with the hand and a strip cup or plate to examine foremilk is a valuable aid in detecting mastitis.
- **Wash teats with solution or pre-dip teats.**

    Only the teats should be washed and then dried. Milking wet udders and teats increases the risk of mastitis.
- **Attach milking units within two minutes**

    Attaching machines within two minutes after first stimulation makes maximum use of the letdown effect. Most cows milk out in five to ten minutes.
- **Adjust units as necessary for proper alignment.**

    Observe units and help prevent liner slips. Minimize irritation and blockage to milk flow. Pay special attention toward the end of the milking to avoid retrograde flow.
- **Ensure vacuum shut-off before removing units.**

    The risk of liner slips and possible new infection is greatest during over-milking. But *how* the teat cups are removed is more important than *when*.
- **Dip teats immediately after unit removal.**

    Use a commercial antiseptic product after every milking. This dramatically reduces the rate of infections.

QUALITY TESTING

The production and processing of high quality milk, with low bacterial count, good flavor and appearance, good keeping qualities and high nutritive value, is ensured in the industry. This is made possible through the co-operative efforts of the dairy farmer, dairy processor, and government departments responsible for enforcing dairy regulations. A number of different tests are made regularly, so computerized records of the quality of milk produced on each farm are generally kept. Most tests are made on milk samples sent to a central government laboratory. In some locations, some tests may be carried out at the farm, and others at the processing plant. In all cases, the procedures and apparatus used in all tests must conform to rigorous government standards.

Composite milk samples from each farm are tested for milk fat at regular intervals usually twice monthly. These are made up of the samples taken by the tank truck driver. Special samples are taken at frequent intervals for other quality tests. **Whenever a batch of milk fails to meet the government standards, it is immediately discarded and the farmer at fault is notified that the quality of his milk supply is below acceptable levels, so he may correct the cause expeditiously.** Regular reports on each farmer's milk supply are filed with the government department responsible for enforcing quality regulations. Most farmers keep records of the amount and quality of milk produced by *each* cow. This information is used for selective breeding and upgrading the herd.

Laboratory Tests
* **Infrared Milk Analysis (IRMA)** is an electronic method of milk analysis used to measure protein, lactose (milk sugar) and milk fat. A beam of infrared light is passed through a very thin film of the milk sample as it flows through a special electric cell. Each milk component absorbs a specific amount of infrared energy at a specific wave length. By electronics, the instrument reads and transposes the amounts of absorbed energy into milk fat, protein and lactose percentages. Direct connection with a computer provides readings in less than one minute.

- **Bacteria Counts** reveal the number of bacteria present in the milk sample, and serve as indicators of milk quality. The test counts the total viable bacteria in a milliliter (ml) of milk. *The Standard Data Count (SDC)* is an indicator of sanitation in milking cows, milking systems cleanup and certain types of mastitis. Quality milk has a count below 5,000. The factors affecting SPC are the level of herd mastitis, high numbers of late lactation cows, milker employee hygiene, cow and milking system cleanliness, milking equipment rubber parts condition and faulty milk pump seal.

  The Laboratory Pasteurized Count (LPC) counts the bacteria that survive pasteurization which affect the flavor and shelf life of the milk. These counts are below 750/ml and may be as low as 50/ml. They are due mainly to poor equipment cleanup and milk residues in the pipeline, traps and tanks. High LPC is not related to mastitis. *Coliform counts (CC)* count the fecal bacteria in milk and coli organisms shed by cows into milk. Again these counts should be below 750/ml and may be as low as 50/ml. The CC value is affected by milking wet and dirty cows and occasionally from defective milking system cleanup. Disinfectant and hot water washing should minimize the latter. Mastitis can elevate the count but very rarely contributes. Even fresh, clean milk will contain small numbers of harmless, milk-souring bacteria. If milk contains undesirable bacteria, it is rejected for human consumption.

- **Inhibitor Tests** determine the presence or absence of antibiotics and pesticides in a milk sample. If these are present, the milk is not accepted.

- **Freezing Point of Milk Test** determines the water content of the milk sample using an apparatus known as a cryoscope. This test discourages any attempt to dilute the milk supply.

- **Somatic cell count or Milk gel index** is a test made on a milk sample to detect the presence of mastitis. Mastitis may be subclinical and not visible in the herd or in individual cows. Counts above 200,000/ml reduce both cow production and the yield and shelf life of the processed product. Suspect cows are removed from the main herd and treated. Possible sources of mastitis include other infected cows, late lactation cows, growth hormone, bedding and corral conditions, milking procedures and equipment failure.

It is trendy (if not popular) to be skeptical about the entire food supply. As was pointed out earlier, with the impact of modern technology, what used to be agricultural food *per se*, has now become in a sense industrial food. And there is ample evidence to demonstrate real issues pertaining to nutritional values and contamination even with respect to staple foods. Studies in women for example, have demonstrated the presence of pesticides in human breast milk. That is cause for serious concern, especially with the high incidence of cancer and disorders in the immune system.

Yet having said that, it is still a far cry to pin the responsibility for poisons in the food supply on dairy farmers or the dairy industry as a whole. The evidence is just not there. Any lactating animal would excrete toxins through her milk if they were present in the blood at the time. This could, in principle at least, include antibiotics, pesticides, chemicals and hormones. Traces of these are permissible under the government standards but only very minute traces! Farmers and veterinarians understand the nature of the problem and also understand the economic costs of any rejection and penalties for contaminated samples. Careful precautions to avoid these are therefore taken. Yes, the animals do get treated when necessary. This includes routine immunizations against specific diseases, the use of antibiotics for infections (particularly mastitis) and even prophylaxis in some areas of the U.S. The use of hormones to increase lactation has been approved in the U.S. but rejected in Canada and Europe. Some types of breeding problems with artificial insemination and associated with irregular cycles, have been connected with naturally-occurring progesterone. Steroids are sometimes used therapeutically as anti-inflammatory drugs.

Of all the dozens of drugs that veternairans use in treating cows, only four (4) are tested for on a routine basis. **Spot tests** in different areas have found some isolated evidences of contamination. The Centre for Science in the Public Interest and The Wall Street Journal (Dec. 29, 1989) reported for example that 38% of milk samples in 10 cities were found to be contaminated with sulfur drugs or other antibiotics. The Nutrition Action Health Letter (1990) reported a 20% contamination rate in a similar study. Yet routine tests by the FDA have repeatedly found levels of such contaminants *below* acceptable standard levels. There may be debate regarding what is an acceptable level for antibiotics, bacteria or pesticides, but clearly the absence of direct clinical evidence in terms of implications to human health would seem to negate the serious concerns raised by dairy antagonists. But constant vigilance is prudent.

On the farm we are visiting today, **antibiotics** are not used prophylactically but only when indication for infection. When infection does occur, the affected animal is clearly identified with visible red markings, as well as electronically to trigger the computer if there were any attempt to collect milk into the same common lines in the milking parlor. The treated animals are tested repeatedly before they re-enter the normal milking line rotation. In the U.S., where the use of antibiotics is more widespread, there are frequent assays to minimize the levels of antibiotics in the milk going to the dairy. Contamination is very costly and that constrains the farmer to follow good farming practices.

Nevertheless, concerned citizens and other activists who berate the dairy industry make consistent accusations. Almost half of all the antibiotics (some 15 million pounds each year) manufactured in the United States are poured directly into animal feeds. The most commonly used ones are penicillin and tetracycline. This excessive use of antibiotics has implications for human health more indirectly because it certainly contributes to *the emergence of new strains of bacteria with antibiotic-resistance*. This has become indeed a major material crisis in public health in North America and all efforts should be mounted now to minimize such liberal use of antibiotics even if economics would dictate otherwise. The argument has been advanced that it is the impact of technology and the factory farm with its confinement practices which has created a breeding ground for infectious diseases and a source of major stress which depletes the animals' immune system. But modern trends in urbanization and declining manpower in farm production makes any return to old-fashioned, family style farming impractical and unnecessary. Solutions must be found for modern farmers to limit their use of antibiotics and other drugs and all other chemical interventions on the farm to reduce the threat to an absolute minimum.

Perhaps the most controversial issue in the dairy industry today, is the use of **Bovine Growth Hormone (BGH)** (or more exactly, Bovine Somatotropin, BST). This is a genetically engineered hormone which upon injection, artificially manipulates lactation in cows to increase milk production by up to 20 percent. It is produced by extracting normal growth hormone from cows, and then using sophisticated gene-splitting techniques to create synthetic hormones which are then injected into dairy cows in many parts of the United States. This is not the place to discuss the details of this practice but both the science, the ethics and the economics have been called into question. The industry claims that the innovation is safe and effective and has gained FDA approval. But others seriously question the approval process which has been fraught with more than political irony from beginning to end. For a detailed discussion of the evidence and the legal dog fight, see '*MILK the Deadly Poison*' by Robert Cohen. More importantly, serious concerns have been raised about the implications – both for the animals and for human health. The particular worry (among others) is that BGH-milk contains higher levels of a human growth promotant and probable carcinogen known as Insulin-like Growth Factor One (IGF –1). Other effects in cows lead to increased mastitis and other sickness, and the use of more antibiotics and other drugs, leading to further possible contamination of the milk supply. This is a hot political and inflammatory issue and readers interested in the on-going debate and political lobbying are advised to pursue this on the Internet or elsewhere.

On the opposite extreme to gene manipulation, **organic farming** systems do not use any toxic chemical pesticides or fertilizers. Instead they are based on the development of biological diversity and the maintenance and replenishment of soil fertility. When certified, a thorough inspection has been done to prove that all procedures satisfy strict uniform standards. Organic livestock are not given antibiotics, hormones or medications (other than vaccinations) applied in the absence of illness. They are given wormers and similar products derived from natural product sources. Livestock diseases and parasites are controlled through preventive measures such as rotational grazing. These organic farmers represent less than 10% of the industry.

On a typical farm, farmers are now giving more thought to withholding periods for grazing after spraying a pasture with weeds, and after spot-spraying for woody weed control. They are also paying more attention to the choice of chemicals - based on the withholding period and the suitability for dairy pastures and crops. They are buying only quality-assured feeds because again the economic costs are high.

BREEDING

In order to make milk, a cow must first have a calf. This first happens when she is about two years old. Then dedicated dairy cows have a calf each year for three to five years. The average length of time a cow gives milk is about three-and-a-half years, after which she is sacrificed at the beef market.

The annual cycle begins at the birth of a young calf. In the dairy we are visiting today, there is a separate maternity wing with ten specially designed stalls and two adjacent nursery rooms each housing four comfortable calf-stalls in a controlled environment. Cows have a normal gestation period of about 280 days (similar to humans) and for the normal pregnancy the cow is milked up to two months before delivery. Then she enters the dry period before being taken off to the maternity barn in preparation for her delivery. There she has a more comfortable environment with larger stalls, well padded floors, and generous access to her feeding trough and water station. Farmers clearly understand the economic value of each new healthy calf and does everything necessary to deliver and care for it. Late in pregnancy, the expectant 'mother' experiences marked weight gain and spends more time lying and resting. In an uncomplicated delivery, the cow becomes more restless and occasionally moans but she can often deliver on her own. Occasionally with a difficult lie or presentation, or with multiple births the farmer or veterinarian is required to assist the delivery. Sometimes cesarean sections are done under local anaesthetic and the loss of either mother or calf is rather rare. In the maternity barn today we have six healthy cows: two have recently given birth, one of which had twins and four are in anticipation of imminent labor. There's usually a veterinarian on call.

At birth, each calf is carefully identified, coded and registered in the appropriate registry. It wears a transponder and a collar from then on. Soon after birth the calf is taken to the nursery for special care. It is fed with colostrum by bottle within hours. Outside 24 hours the calf cannot use colostrum efficiently and without it, its chance of survival is much reduced. This special pre-milk or early milk is critical for maternal antibodies especially, to pass to the calf for its protection immediately after birth. Colostrum is stored in a freezer here on this farm for use when necessary for whatever reason. The calf remains in the nursery for about 3-4 months during which period it gets special care.

Breeding has become a high-tech area of farming since genetic engineering has allowed the selection of the best dairy cows in terms of general health and obviously, milk production. Strange as it may seem, *computer dating* where particular bulls are crossed with their chosen partners is now more the rule than the exception.

Pregnancy is induced by artificial insemination. The technicians on the farm are each skilled in inserting the arm and then, using an 8"-10" long stainless steel tube all covered in plastic, he takes the frozen semen sample (all computer coded by semen suppliers) and loads 'the gun'. When he finds his place, he skillfully fires and hopes for the best. Sometimes it may require two or three attempts but it is usual to inseminate once each year about three months after the last calf, while the heifer is still on her daily milking routine.

It is simply amazing how productive these cows can be. And yes, they are exploited to the maximum. After all, more than 90 percent of the milk each cow produces goes to feed humans and less than ten percent is utilized by its intended beneficiary – her young baby calf. That milk goes to the dairy where it is then processed and treated to provide a range of dairy products designed to appeal to every segment of the human market.

MILK PRODUCTS

Milk has been exploited as a raw material in the manufacture of complete lines of dairy products to satisfy consumer needs and tastes. These include beverages, creams, concentrates, cultured foods, ice creams, cheese and butter. They vary in both nutritional content and potential health consequences, but in practice they are all basically products for sale – subject to the same marketing forces as any other commercial offering. Therefore, it is still wise to observe: *caveat emptor* – buyer beware.

Standards for the composition of milk are established by the government to keep the ingredients constant, since they do vary with the individual cow, the breed of cow and the season. Milk is standardized at each processing plant by pooling the tested and screened production batches from several farms at a time. Almost all jurisdictions in North America require that milk sold to the consumer be pasteurized and be so labeled.

Fresh Fluid Milks

Whole milk is defined as milk that contains at least 3.25% milk fat and at least 8% non-fat milk solids. Most of the fluid whole milk marketed is homogenized. When some of the fat in milk is removed, it is called partly skimmed milk, partially skimmed milk or low fat milk, depending on the area in which it is sold. Standards for fat content vary from 0.17 to 3.2% milk fat, but the most common product contains two percent fat and is called *2% MILK*. All partially skimmed milk is homogenized. *Skim milk*, or skimmed milk, usually refers to milk which has had most of the fat removed. The residual level of fat in skim milk is about 1%. Sterilized milk (*UHT milk*) is milk which has been heated to a temperature of 100°C to destroy all organisms present and is packaged in hermetically sealed containers. It contains not less than 3.25% milk fat.

Creams

Cream is made by separating standard milk into skim milk and cream containing about 40% milk fat. This concentrated cream is diluted with milk to obtain fat levels as follows: *Light cream* (cereal cream) may contain 8 to 15.9% fat, but is usually 10% fat by weight; *half and half* contains 8 to 15.9% fat, but has about 11.5% fat and has 8 to 15.9% non-fat solids; *table cream*, often called "cream", usually is 18% but may have 16 to 31.9% fat; *whipping cream* usually contains 35% fat, but ranges from 30 to 35%, and when packed in aerosol cans, it may range from 18 to 26%. Regulations usually permit a "pH adjusting agent" in fresh cream, and if indicated on the label, a stabilizing agent such as sodium citrate. The stabilizer helps prevent the feathery flakes that may form when cream is added to hot liquids.

Sterilized cream (*UHT cream*) is homogenized cream heated to 140.5°C and held, under pressure, at that temperature for 2 seconds. It is then cooled rapidly to 70°C, the pressure released, cooled again to

15.6°C and packaged aseptically. It is then cooled to 4.44°C. Unopened, this cream will keep for several weeks at room temperature. Once the package is opened, the cream must be refrigerated.

Specially Processed Milks

Some milks are flavored, essentially for taste. Examples are *chocolate milk* which must contain at least 3% milk fat, and chocolate partially skimmed milk which must contain greater than 0.1% and less than 3% fat. Chocolate or cocoa, a sweetening agent, and sometimes salt, are added to whole or partially skimmed milk.

Modified milks are identified as skim milk and partially skimmed milk, with added milk solids containing not less than 10% milk solids. Skim milk powders and/or evaporated milk are used to provide the milk solids.

Some beverages made from a milk base do not qualify as milk under formal regulations. They are non-standardized products. Examples include powdered chocolate beverage, eggnog and instant breakfast.

Concentrated Milks

Powdered whole milk and powdered skim milk are powdered milks with about 3% water content. Most powdered milk is made by the spray-dry process, in which partly evaporated milk is sprayed into a heated chamber where it dries almost instantly and falls as a powder ready for cooling, sifting and packaging. Powdered whole milk must be packaged in a vacuum as an extra precaution to prevent the oxidation of fat. To produce "instantized" skim milk powder that readily dissolves, the skim milk powder is blown into a chamber containing air saturated with steam, where the minute particles aggregate into larger particles containing many tiny air spaces. Dry buttermilk, containing a maximum of 5% moisture and at least 4.5% milk fat, is processed primarily for commercial use.

Evaporated milk, sometimes called concentrated milk, includes evaporated whole, evaporated partly skimmed and evaporated skim milks, depending on the type of milk used in its production. All have a darker color than the original milk because at high temperatures a browning reaction occurs between the milk protein and the lactose. In processing, the milk is standardized to a desired ratio of solids to fat and forewarmed to prevent the casein from coagulating during sterilization. After 60% of the water is removed by evaporation, the milk is homogenized, cooled, restandardized and canned. Then it is sterilized by heating for 10 to 15 minutes at 98.9° to 120°C. Controlled amounts of disodium phosphate and/or sodium citrate preserve the "salt balance" and prevent coagulation of the milk that might occur at high temperatures and during storage.

Sweetened *condensed milk* is a viscous, sweet, cream colored milk made by condensing milk to 1/3 of its original volume to which sugar has been added. It contains about 40% sugar, a minimum of 8.5% milk fat and 28% total milk solids. High temperatures of evaporation pasteurize the milk and its high sugar content acts as a preservative, making sterilization unnecessary.

Malted milk is a powdered product containing at least 7.5% milk fat and not more than 3.5% moisture. Malt is added to whole milk and the mixture is dehydrated after the enzymatic action of the malt is completed.

Cultured Dairy Foods

Cultured dairy foods are prepared by adding bacterial cultures to pasteurized or sterilized milk to convert the lactose into lactic acid, the citric acid into diacetyl; and to coagulate the casein. These products include yogurt, sour cream (salad cream), buttermilk and cottage cheese.

Yogurt is a delicate, tangy product made from either whole milk, partly skimmed milk or skim milk (with skim milk powder sometimes added) to make a total of about 16% milk solids. Although it ranges from 1 to 3% milk fat, yogurt usually contains 2% fat. It is available as the plain milk product or with added flavorings (fruit or vanilla), fruit or fruit juice. Yogurt is made by heating pasteurized, homogenized milk to suitable temperatures and inoculating it with acid producing bacterial cultures. If a set custard type (a semi-solid consistency) is desired, the warm inoculated milk is put directly into consumer containers, incubated under controlled conditions, then cooled to less than 4.44°C. When these yogurts contain fruit, the fruit mixture is layered in the bottom of the container before the milk preparation is added. In making the stirred type (Swiss style), the vats of warm inoculated milk are incubated, cooled to less than 4.44°C and stored for up to 48 hours. Then it is stirred to a smooth, cream-like consistency and the fruit preparation is added. Yogurt has a storage life of 2 to 4 weeks when properly refrigerated. Yogurt drinks are processed in a similar manner to yogurt to provide a tangy beverage. The fat content of the drinks varies according to the manufacturer.

Buttermilk has a characteristic tangy flavor, a smooth rich body and contains from 0.1 to 2% milk fat. Originally, it was a by-product of butter-making. Today it is made by the culture method...the controlled fermentation of lactic acid and flavor-producing bacteria. Buttermilk is produced from pasteurized skim milk fortified with skimmed milk solids, or from partly skimmed milk to which milk fat is added in the form of homogenized cream. Milk is inoculated with the culture, incubated under controlled conditions until 0.8 to 0.9% acidity is reached; then cooled quickly to 10°C at which time salt may be added for flavor. Sour cream has a delicate aromatic flavor and contains from 10 to 18% milk fat by weight. This cultured milk product is made by the same process as buttermilk, by ripening pasteurized cream with a lactic acid culture.

Frozen Dairy Foods

Ice cream contains at least 36% total solids, at least 10% of which is milk fat in most flavors. In the case of added chocolate, fruit, nuts, etc., the amount of fat may be proportionately reduced to a minimum of 8%. One of the most popular of a number of frozen dairy products, is made from a mix, which is a combination of basic ingredients. These include cream, whole and/or condensed milk, and/or other milk solids, sugar (a portion of which may be corn sugar or glucose) and flavoring. A stabilizer of vegetable origin and an emulsifier, which together may take up not more than 0.5% of the mix, are also added. The mix is pasteurized, homogenized, flavored if desired and then frozen rapidly to obtain a smooth, creamy product. During freezing, air is incorporated by whipping to provide the increase in volume (known as "overrun") that is essential for a light, desirable product. Most commonly the overrun is 80 to 110%. After packaging, ice cream is hardened at -31°C and held at −23.9 to 28.9°C during storage and distribution. Soft ice cream, a smooth, compact product with at least 8 to 10% milk fat, has slightly more non-fat solids and 2 to 3% less sugar than hard ice cream. The extra milk solids, the stabilizers and emulsifiers used, the overrun of about 40% and the serving temperature of –6.67 to 7.78°C, all contribute to its soft texture.

Ice milk contains between 3 to 5% milk fat and 33% total solids. Made from milk, it contains added milk solids, sugar and flavoring, and has an average overrun of 90%. In its soft form, it sometimes is sold as soft ice cream. *Sherbet* is a tart flavored product with a maximum of 5% total milk solids, and an overrun of 30 to 35%. Fresh or dried skim milk and milk fat, added to a base of syrup and fruit juice, constitute its basic ingredients. Frozen yogurt, as the name implies, is a frozen version of yogurt. A stabilizer and flavoring may be added.

Cheese

There are many different types of cheeses, both natural and processed. Several factors determine their distinctive flavor, texture and appearance: the kinds of milk used, the method for setting the curd, the type of bacteria used in ripening, the temperature and humidity during ripening, the length of time the cheese is aged, and the amount of salt or other seasonings added. All natural cheeses are made from milk, cream or whey.

Cheddar is probably the most famous of natural-type cheeses and is produced in greater quantity than any other. Most cheddars are made from pasteurized cow's milk, but the highest quality cheddar is generally made from raw milk. The process involves heating the milk to 30.6°C, putting in a starter to promote the growth of lactic acid-forming organisms, then adding rennet to form the curd. The curd is heated to 37.6°C, then the whey is drained off and salt added. After cutting, the curd is compressed into large forms and held at 14.4 to 15.6°C for at least 8 days. The cheese is reopened or cured at 4.44 to 10.0°C for varying lengths of time…one year for "old", at least 6 months for "medium" and at least 60 days for "mild" cheddar. Sixty days is the minimum time required to destroy any harmful bacteria that might be present. During the ripening process, the characteristic cheddar flavor and body are developed. The longer the ripening period, the sharper and nippier the flavor, and the softer the texture. When coloring is added, the cheese becomes a deep orange shade rather than its natural cream color.

Cottage cheese, another type, is a fresh, soft, milk white cheese.

It is made by adding a lactic acid-producing starter, and a coagulator such as rennet, to pasteurized skim milk, either fresh or reconstituted. The resulting curd is cut and heated to develop texture and body, then the whey is removed and the curd is washed. Salt may be added. Small curd and large curd cottage cheese are both solid, either dry or creamed. In the latter, a blend of pasteurized cream and dry curd makes a product with at least 4% milk fat by weight. Fruits, vegetables, spices and herbs may be added.

Cream cheese, also a fresh cheese, has a mild flavor and contains a higher proportion of moisture and fat than other natural cheeses. It is made from cream, or a blend of milk and cream, with flavoring and seasoning often added for variety. Whey cheeses, such as ricotta, are made by using heat and acid to coagulate the protein in the whey recovered from other cheese-making processes.

As well as the previously mentioned cheeses, there are dozens of additional natural variety cheeses commercially available. Each has its own distinctive flavor and texture and is manufactured under carefully controlled conditions. *Processed cheeses* are really a blend of natural cheeses. These are ground, melted and pasteurized then blended with one or more optional ingredients: milk solids, water, coloring agents, seasonings, relishes, emulsifiers and preservatives. While hot, the semi-liquid mixture is poured into molds, jars or packages.

Butter

Butter is a product made from cream. In addition to the minimum 80% by weight from fat, it contains milk solids, usually some salt (sweet butter contains no added salt) and coloring may be added. It is manufactured either by the churning method, or by the continuous method which gives butter a slightly different texture. Both methods use sweet, neutralized or ripened cream, pasteurized and standardized to a usual fat content of 30 to 40%.

That was just a brief outline, indicative of the variety of dairy foods. The modern supermarket has thousands of other items that invite the consumer to make choices. That's where you the reader, will come in. You must make wise decisive lifestyle choices that will generate both a healthy body and a healthy mind. To that end, the last chapter of this review of nature's goldmine is dedicated to give you some practical tips on making the necessary healthy lifestyle choices. You will learn to eat well and feel good.

Chapter Twelve

EAT WELL, FEEL GOOD

We began in Chapter One with a peek into the Alternative Medicine and Wellness Arena. We pointed out that much of this is a reaction to the dramatic advances in modern science and medicine which unfortunately, have still left us with much chronic illness. In addition, this specialized knowledge has reduced the patient into a collection of specialized body parts. Contemporary clinical practice with its sophisticated diagnostics, its plethora of new wonder medications, and its advanced surgical techniques, has virtually left the patient out of his or her own management and care. For these reasons and more, the public has made a major shift in its healthcare perspectives and is turning more and more back to nature, back to the traditional and unconventional healing arts.

But we have advanced the position throughout this book that the most promising way forward in health is at the *interface* of nature and science. This was so clearly illustrated in Chapters Four, Five and Six by the serendipitous discovery of Dr. Bounous and his colleagues. They found, in something as natural as whey (and breast milk), the bioactive proteins that can deliver the rate-limiting precursors to modulate intracellular glutathione. This advance is even more revealing, now that we are discovering further implications of glutathione's function in cell-defense and in the immune response. This is a unique secret of nature, now revealed by good science. Or who would have imagined that the unusual benzodiazepine-type receptor site in the GABA-chloride-ionophore-receptor complex of the most prevalent inhibitory neurotransmitter in the central nervous system, would fit like hand in glove with an enzyme hydrolysis product of a major milk protein. Chapters Seven, Eight and Nine told this amazing story. Again, it is **the designs**

of nature being uncovered by the devices of science. It is like mining for gold in nature and finding a healthy treasure.

When we strip away all the philosophies and rhetoric of the Wellness advocates – there seems to be at least two dominant foci for their concerns. The first is for the individual person to take more responsibility for their own health and care, and so to make a number of critical decisions in terms of lifestyle and personal management. This leads to the reclaiming of personal autonomy and real significance. It puts the control of one's life where it truly belongs – in one's own hands. The second focus is on the quality of life – in its totality. Health is seen then in the broadest possible terms as a harmony of physical, psychological, social and spiritual factors leading to a state of personal rest, freedom from pain, and a sense of fulfillment. It is a product of choice as much as chance.

You remember Rick and Celeste? They were our yuppie couple from Chapter One. They were making choices – from all appearances, some healthy choices. Wellness was indeed their goal. They wanted the best that life had to offer and so Health was Job One. They knew it would not happen by accident or osmosis. It would be a result of them taking responsibility, becoming aware of their options and exercising direction and discipline. *You* should do no less. You too, should take responsibility for your own health. You should explore all your options and make the right decisions.

Of all the lifestyle choices you will make on a daily basis, the choice of what you eat is paramount, if you do at all believe with Adelle Davis, that 'we are what we eat'. As your body turns over by cell renewal, your genetics will dictate much of the course of physical change, but you at least have some control of the raw material input. This is an ordinary activity of human nature and should be dominated by the consumption of natural rather than industrial food. We will shortly outline a decalogue of instructions for you to do this with maximum efficiency and for the benefit of your healthy body's future.

Similarly, in an age when your health is threatened by the toxins and pollutants in the environment and by the incessant pressures and hectic demands of modern existence, rife with change and uncertainty, there are strategies for coping from which you can benefit. These will be explored to your advantage in the second half of this final chapter.

The net result should be a relief from anxiety and a discovery of a new quality of life that derives from an inward tranquility of mind, a fortified immunity of body and combined together, a renewed *vim and vigor* that creates for you an improved quality of life for years to come.

TEN COMMANDMENTS OF GOOD NUTRITION

Commandment #1   Eat Small, Regular and Varied Meals

North Americans eat too much. In our affluence, with so many consumer products and with the ubiquitous advertising that manipulates our appetites and decisions, we can't seem to get enough to put into our mouths. We want to satisfy those taste buds for everything that 'tastes great' but 'works bad', and to fill our bloated stomachs to capacity. Whether it's 'death by chocolate' or late night pizzas, or those huge 16oz steaks from off the grill, or any of the myriad of treats and tantalizing recipes that keep growing in number, we just can't resist the urge to keep up the pace of food consumption. And we pay dearly for it all.

The consequence is an obese population. More than 60 million North American adults (approximately one-third of that population) between the ages of 20 and 74 are considered overweight (obese). And this despite the unending stream of diet books and weight-loss programs that offer magic solutions to get rid of those unwanted pounds. It is both a vanity issue and a health issue. Whatever the reason, keeping the weight off is the way to go. If indeed we are serious about health and wellness, we have no choice but to wisely reduce our consumption of empty calories and particularly high fat content.

Unlike some other animals, we have relatively small stomachs designed for small, frequent meals. As rational and intelligent creatures who should operate more on brain function than on brute force, diverting blood flow continuously to aid digestion is counter-productive. We're a long way from survival in the jungle. So let's be discreet, cut back on meal portions and eat smaller meals.

In a fast-paced society with increased responsibility and expectations, our daily schedules often dictate our lives. Hence, a pronounced shift to fast, convenience and junk foods. For far too many, eating is an interruption in their daily routines. So many try to get by on a donut and coffee for breakfast (if at all), a fast food lunch eaten on the run (when time permits) and then a packaged dinner warmed over in the micro-wave. That is no nutritious way to go. But whenever such people get hungry, there's something sweet, fatty and tasty to fill their aching stom-ach. With over 300,000 fast food restaurants in the U.S., they have become an integral part of the busy American lifestyle. Too often that implies food high in calories, sodium, fat and cholesterol. It tends to feed our taste buds and our stomachs, but often starves our bodies.

With changing family structures and styles, the nutritional needs tend to be neglected. The family dining room has just about gone out with the Women's Movement and meal times no longer exist. So eating has become erratic and often impulsive. The result is the same: a trend to fast, convenience and junk foods. We eat as it were anytime, over-time and sometimes at no-time. But if we are to regain control of our health status, we must adopt new lifestyle patterns to include small, regular and nutritious meals.

Variety is the key to a nutritious diet. You need not worry about all the Food Group classifications and the diet charts. A basic rule of thumb is to practice the *Rainbow Diet*. Each meal should reflect as much as possible, the colors of the rainbow in all its diversity. This would certainly shift food choices to include more of the essential (but neglected) fresh fruits and vegetables, plus wholesome cereals and grains. These make great snack foods too. You could have a ball enjoying the delights of nature on about 2000 calories/day and still feel satisfied and energized.

Adelle Davis was right. You will become what you eat. So food choice and dietary habit are indeed crucial in the pursuit of the best of health and all that life has to offer. So this is a great place to begin: with small, regular and varied meals. Choose wisely.

Commandment #2   Drink 6 – 8 Glasses of Fluid each Day

Adequate fluid intake is a necessary healthy habit. Our bodies are living, active, regenerating machines made up of 50-60 percent wa-ter. The end product of metabolism is to produce non-toxic waste which is discarded principally by urinary output. On a daily basis, a normal healthy adult loses about 1500 ml of water as urine, 500 ml through skin evaporation, about 400 ml in normal respiration and finally, about 200ml in feces. This all adds up to about 2.6 litres of fluid loss each day. This needs to be replaced by at least six glasses of fluid of one kind or another. The body can easily handle even more by increasing urinary output through kidney control. If we happen to drink less, the lower volume of urine becomes more concentrated, assuming the kidney can cope with the additional stress.

Fluids represent a very large market and so beverages and drinks of all kinds have been a major component of advertising. The legendary rise of Atlanta's Coca Cola Company has made that soft drink a household name around the world. In more recent times, the head-to-head competition with rival Pepsi has helped to sustain the consumption of carbonated soft drinks across the board. Alcoholic beverages, with the rise of competitive sports and associated beer advertising, has continued to hold market share and shows no signs of declining. Hot beverages have their own place in the market and the stunning success of Starbucks in the U.S. and Tim Hortons in Canada illustrates the place of coffee in modern culture. And that's where many people turn for their fluid intake: soft drinks, alcoholic beverages and coffee. They each have associated problems which are well known. Soft drinks are usually full of empty calories and food additives and deplete some valuable nutrients; alcohol abuse has a myriad of personal and social consequences (even without spouse abuse and drunk driving); and coffee is known to contain the active caffeine ingredient with physiological effects that show a related dose response. So although copious fluid intake is essential and makes a lot of sense, the choice of what to drink each day is not without consequences.

What should you be drinking as a habit? The answer is a combination of pure water, fruit juices and yes, some refreshing milk if you can tolerate it. *Pure* water is specified because water quality in many jurisdictions across North America has been rightfully brought into question in small towns and communities, as well as in large cities. The public has been losing faith in the authorities' claim of pure drinking water, questioning the very standards that are used. The not infrequent media reports of water-borne illnesses from bacterial contamination and so on, does not do anything to reassure the public. The increasing use of bottled water may be a good trend, although in some cases it is questionable if one is being sold genuine water purity or just another label. In-home purification with water filters, distillers and reverse osmosis units does make sense in most cases. The increasing trend to just drinking water at home, on the job and even in restaurants is a healthy one.

Fruit juices make good nutritional sense. When obtained directly from washed fruits, that is the ideal. Usually rich in Vitamin C and all the benefits to be derived from that, there is the conspicuous absence of additives for flavor and taste. Natural is best in this regard. Fruit *drinks* (contrasted with juices) are packaged and advertised to mislead the public. These are usually not rich in nutrients, and often contain an abundance of chemical additives that can only do more harm than good. The *power* drinks, so well promoted by high performance athletes and almost saturating media sports, are more hype than nutritional substance. Endurance athletes who experience extensive electrolyte losses, can benefit from electrolyte replacement available in some of these preparations, but the normal individual in a typical daily routine has little to gain from them.

Milk completes this fluid triad. Dairy promoters would like us all to consume 3, 4 or even 5 glasses of milk daily. We would be wiser to be more restrained given at least the incidence of lactose or milk protein intolerance and the high fat content of whole milk. But all things in moderation. Milk as a beverage is appropriate but not indispensable for many in the population. It makes a nutritious contribution to a balanced and adequate North American diet.

Commandment #3   Reduce Salt and Refined Sugar

Eating preserved and processed foods has become a way of life in North America. It is almost impossible to prepare a meal even at home, without using some processed food. Seventy five percent of the sodium we consume is in those processed foods. What the food industry included during processing, we just can't take out. So even if we reduce our salt intake, that won't solve the problem. But we should do what we can.

The human body needs salt to function. Sodium is the main component of the body's extracellular fluids and it helps carry nutrients into the cells. Sodium also helps regulate other body functions, especially blood pressure. The National Research Council of the National Academy of Sciences in Washington D.C., recommended daily intake of 500-2400 mg of sodium, preferably below 1800mg. Many Americans are consuming much higher amounts, up to 6000 mg/day. This excess is eliminated by healthy kidneys but at the expense of the accompanying calcium loss.

High intake of salt over time produces physiological changes in the kidney, increasing the risk of hypertension and its complications. More than 50 million North Americans have clinical hypertension so this is no light matter. Too much salt seems to overwork the sodium channels in the kidney and the process is irreversible. Therefore, it is more than prudent to restrict salt intake. Simple lifestyle adjustments become necessary and it does not take long to adjust to more neutral tastes.

So, take stock of the sources of salt in your diet. Read the labels on foods. Ask chefs to omit salt where necessary. Use more high potassium foods, such as fresh fruits and vegetables. Try new spices and herbs to flavor foods. Finally, if you must salt while cooking (only), add the salt at the end where you will need to add much less.

A similar story applies to sugar. The typical person in North America consumes about 140lb sugar per year. That is a lot of empty calories designed to satisfy one of the four sensuous tastebud categories (salty, sweet, sour and bitter). Most of the sugar is again hidden in our foods and seems to be the *raison d'etre* of many a fast food operation. It adds taste and causes satiety – just what the marketer ordered.

The debate about the impact of high refined-sugar consumption has still not ended. Orthodoxy insists that we are equipped physiologically to handle high sugar loads. But millions testify to changes in mood and behavior not long after a pulse of sweets in the diet. Whether there is a tendency to hypoglycemia in some individuals giving rise to transient (reversible) clinical symptoms may remain controversial. We do know that high refined-sugar diets contribute to dental caries (sweet tooth), that diets high in sugar tend to be low in nutrition across the board, and that the consumption of sugar benefits the normal individual very little, if at all.

So cut back on salt and sugar in your diet.

Commandment #4 **Run From Fat**

Dietary fat and cholesterol have taken a justified heavy beating in the media for the past two decades and more. Most consumers are now aware that high fat consumption contributes to major diseases including heart disease and stroke, some forms of cancer, as well as diabetes and possibly, secondary hypertension. Many public health and nutrition awareness programs have got the message out. So much so that we have seen a distinct trend towards reducing fat consumption. Food manufacturers and marketers are not to be outdone, so they have created a new industry of low-fat foods which have taken over many sections of the neighborhood supermarket such as milk and dairy products, salad dressings, processed meats etc.

The U.S. Departments of Agriculture and Health and Human Services, as well as Health and Welfare Canada, have established dietary guidelines for fat and cholesterol: Adults as a whole should consume no more than 30% of total calories as fat. For active men, that means < 73 gm/day of fat; and for most women and older adults that means < 53 gm/day. Similarly, all groups should restrict cholesterol intake to no more than 300 mg/day. Those at risk for heart disease, hypertension or diabetes should restrict both even further. Surveys show that most people in North America are reducing their fat intake and that's a healthy trend. However, in real terms, we still consume on average, about 34% of total calories as fat and as much as 500-600 mg cholesterol per person each day.

Distinctions have been made between saturated and unsaturated fats. The former tends to clog the arteries while the latter tends to become rancid and introduce free radicals which are potentially lethal to the body. On balance, unsaturated fat is the lesser of the two evils. But evils they both are and therefore to be avoided - with a few possible exceptions. Unsaturated omega-3 and omega-6 fatty acids have been shown to be protective against disease, possibly acting as antioxidants in their own right. These are prevalent in deep sea fish and made available as capsules or oil.

As far as cholesterol goes, there has been a lot of hype and folklore surrounding the importance of this steroid. The body makes all the cholesterol it needs and has a complex recycling mechanism to optimize its valuable functions. Diets high in fat and cholesterol tend to increase the levels of bad (LDL) cholesterol while moderate exercise tends to favor the good (HDL) cholesterol. High blood cholesterol levels increase the risk for heart disease.

Clearly, a low-fat diet is a healthy diet and fat is to be avoided in all forms, at all times, in all places and by all means. It is a dangerous killer. Therefore, take all precautions to minimize your level of fat consumption both at home and away from home. Limit high-fat meats, whole milk and cheese. Choose fish and lean poultry instead. Steam or broil foods, fry and barbecue less. Use vegetable oils rather than fats that are solid at room temperature. Be on guard when eating out for it's your arteries at risk - not the chef's. The jury is still out on fat substitutes.

Commandment #5   Up Your Fiber

Oat bran is here to stay. Unlike so many foods that come and go because they have no real value, the surge in interest and consumption of oat-bran going back two decades was based in good science. Oat bran is a good source of fiber, a dietary component with unique characteristics: it is not digested, absorbed or metabolized by the body. Instead, fiber passes directly through the digestive system and reaches the large intestine as semi-solid mass. Observations on the role of this fiber in the body have given it an important new status in the diet, essentially providing bulk and solvency. It is critical in disease prevention.

Dietary fiber provides this bulk to the digestive tract aiding motility, promoting regularity and easing elimination. It binds cholesterol in the gut and serves to reduce serum levels. It modulates sugar absorption to improve glucose tolerance, particularly for diabetics. It provides satiety after meals, restraining consumption of empty calories and fats, thereby reducing obese tendencies. Finally, dietary fiber is believed to also bind toxins and potential carcinogens in the gut and thereby exerts a protective influence. There is now clear epidemiological association between a high-fiber diet and a reduction in the risk of cardiovascular disease, large bowel cancer, diverticulosis, constipation and other chronic disorders.

But since the invention of the roller mill which allowed mass distribution of soft white flour with most of the cereal and grain fiber removed, fiber consumption plunged and gastrointestinal disorders soared. Around the turn of the century, the average North American ate about 53lbs (24kg) of apples (an excellent source of fiber). Today the average person eats only 20lbs(9kg) or one apple per week. We do not even comply with the overstated adage, 'an apple a day to keep the doctor away'. Fiber intake including whole grains, beans, fresh vegetables and fresh fruit has declined by 50% since 1910, while fat intake has risen 25 percent. The same trend toward fast, convenience and junk foods that we noted earlier, is also responsible for this decline in fiber consumption. Effective marketing and advertising of the highly-processed, chemically-preserved food products that industry now provides, has shifted many consumers food choices away from natural, wholesome fiber-rich nutritious foods, and that's not without consequences.

Dr. Dennis Burkitt who is regarded as the father of the Fiber Revolution in this 'wellness' generation, observed in East Africa where he trained young doctors, the low incidence of gastro- intestinal diseases and was able to establish the correlation with the high fiber consumption in that part of the world. Living in the Industrial West, we would do well to learn similar dietary habits and consciously choose to increase consumption of good sources of fiber: whole grains and cereals (including oat bran); legumes (dry beans, peas, lentils); nuts and seeds; fruits and vegetables with edible skins (apples, peaches, blueberries), broccoli, cabbage, cauliflower, celery, corn; and root vegetables (beets, carrots, sweet potatoes, turnips).

Now you know the score, you know the sources – just ... Up your Fiber, for the health of it!

Commandment #6   **Shop For Health**

The rise in popularity of huge shopping malls and superstores has transformed the style, the frequency and the purchasing habits of consumers in most urban centers. Gone are the milkman and the farmer's market, or the local butcher or fish market. In their place have come these vast consumption shrines with long parallel aisles; colorful attractive displays of thousands of consumer items; busy, stressed-out shoppers pushing overloaded buggies in often congested traffic, buying on impulse every new concoction that marketers and advertisers can bring daily into our living rooms or display under neon lights. This is twenty first century grocery shopping.

Retailers have done their homework. They have used miniature video cameras, heart rate monitors, barcodes, laser scanners and every other conceivable tracking device to study shopping behavior patterns. The psychologists have exploited the information and provided retail marketing companies with weapons to manipulate the consumer into buying what they want, when they want and how they want. Overspending in grocery stores happens through carefully planned store strategies and advertising; supermarkets are able to persuade us inadvertently to consume what they choose for us, based on one single index – profitability. It's their *raison d'etre*.

They greet us with what they choose in 'the power alley' as we enter. Basic necessities are deliberately placed in the opposite or back ends of the establishment, so we must walk through to get them. En route we must use our eyes. Products that sell well are placed on the top or bottom shelves and those they choose for us are displayed at eye level, just at arm's reach. The soft music, the extra halogen track lighting, the baking aromas, the store brand labels, the aisle specials, etc, etc, are all skillfully crafted to manipulate our impulse-buying decisions. Eighty cents of every dollar that is spent in a grocery store is the result of impulse-buying.

In the light of all this, again *caveat emptor*: buyer beware. You will become what you eat and you will eat what you buy. Therefore, be most careful and alert when you *buy* – especially if you have small children or teenagers. They will eat what's taken in the house. Health-watchers and baby boomers intent on maximum wellness like Rick and Celeste, must take back responsibility and overcome impulse buying behavior for the sake of their own health. In the grocery store, health is at the opposite end to convenience and profitability.

Shop for health. Imagine a huge display sign over the entrance of your supermarket "SHOP FOR HEALTH – HERE'S LIFE AND DEATH". Then govern yourself accordingly. Avoid shopping when you're hungry or hurried, and if at all possible, leave small children at home. Make a list before you go – at least to start with. Begin at the fruit and vegetable aisle and just bypass three aisles: the convenience foods, the snack foods, the prepared ready-to-eat foods. Think about fat and fiber, one down and one up. Read food labels. Be prepared to stretch and bend. Check-out without checking-out the check-out displays. Finally and firstly, budget!

Shop for health or else …!

Commandment #7   **Avoid Crash Diets**

Crash diets will make you crash! It's that simple. The irony of modern lifestyles is the tendency to gluttony on one hand and the obsession with stereotype images of slimness and trimness on the other. The only way to have it both ways, as it were, is to eat like a pig some of the time, and then starve yourself in one way or another when the pendulum weigh-scales go too far. It makes no sense, but all behaviors dictated by advertising and hype never do.

The crazy promoters on television, the best-selling authors of diet books, the commercial weight-loss programs that promise dramatic results in record times with minimal effort or change – watch out, they will all leave you flat and frustrated. They could even do more harm. Crash dieters have been known to experience a wide variety of health complications including cardiac disorders, gall bladder damage and even in the extreme, death. It is believed that the physical health risk in people who repeatedly go through huge weight losses followed by weight gains, is likely greater than if they were to stay the same weight above ideal.

Whatever your genetic predisposition may be, whether you subscribe to nature or nurture as the dominating influence in your body weight just now; and whether you favor the arguments about metabolic rates and set-point theory – you can be sure of one thing: crash diets will not solve any weight problem that you may have. Unwanted pounds of fat are the net product of a calorie equation. Calories go in by mouth and calories burn off through metabolism and exercise. The difference is stored, usually as fat and sometimes through design and discipline, as muscle. Water retention in the body tissues is a separate issue.

Sensible weight-loss is always to be gained through a calculated change in lifestyle that reduces calorie intake and increases calorie utilization. Most responsible physiologists advise today an optimum target rate for weight reduction (when necessary) of two to three pounds (one to one-and-a-half kilograms) per week.

Crash diets starve the body of unwanted calories but also of necessary nutrients. Crash diets are unnatural and unsatisfying and therefore poorly maintained indefinitely. Crash diets are manipulative disciplined choices. Crash diets avoid underlying personal and social issues. Crash diets necessitate no fundamental changes. Crash diets are self-defeating. Crash diets are unhealthy. Crash diets fail!

Therefore, Avoid Crash Diets!

Commandment #8   **Fast Briefly, Once Each Week**

Fasting is the voluntary abstinence from solid food over any period of time out of the ordinary. It is not dieting and should not be related to dieting. The thought of decreased quantity of food - not to mention *no food* - over any extended period of time, is enough to strike terror into the hearts of many people. Those addicted to quantity of food must consider any suggestion of fasting to be off the radar screen. But not quite, it does make sense when practiced correctly and it does have its place in modern culture.

The reality is that consistent eating places a consistent stress on the gastrointestinal tract. There is the regular peristaltic motion, the necessary secretion of digestive juices in the early stages and the absorption of digested nutrients in the later stages in the intestines. Finally, there is need for regular elimination of undigested bulk fibers and toxic wastes produced by digestion and bacterial fermentation. The epithelial lining of this 40' column from end to end is subject to all types of chemical and physical stress, and needs constant renewal and overhaul. Oral hygiene on the front end is common universal practice. Harsh or aggressive colonic treatments at the distal end are at best controversial and at worst, dangerous. In between, the occasional single use of laxatives (perhaps annually) is an effective mode of spring cleaning the inner environment. Nature provides a spontaneous physiological mechanism by the movement of fine cilia hairs that act with epithelial secretions along the walls, to brush and renew the gut lining systematically. But we consume food so fast, so frequently and so fully, that it is prudent to occasionally take a break, give the system a rest and let nature renew the course. This of course, is one function of the diurnal cycle of work and sleep. During the night, there is renewal and cleansing of many organ systems. But large fatty meals, late night snacking and the stress of late night television do not aid the process.

You could benefit from a simple, minor fast routine. Choose one night in the week, preferably Friday or Saturday (with the weekend following) and after a light supper in the early evening, have nothing by mouth but water until lunch time or even supper time the next day. This gives the gut an 18-24 hour rest during which, with the aid of clear fluids, it can undergo restorative cleansing on a regular basis.

This is not recommended for diabetics and hypoglycemic patients whose glucose tolerance is limited. Neither is this suggested for those who are constitutionally unwell, or for small children.

The meal that follows this brief suggested fast should be a light snack of simple foods. This brief fasting period is not the ideal time for undertaking major demanding tasks or to elicit unnecessary stress. It is to be re-creative, restful and refreshing.

Go ahead and try it. Your gut will thank you and you may be spared some discomfort and morbidity later.

Commandment #9   **Treat Yourself**

Eating is a necessity but it should also be a pleasure. A healthy diet must invariably be a fun diet, or else it is not a true diet but a self-inflicted punishment. Whatever limitations you arrive at – whether restricting calories, reducing fat, avoiding junk food, eating at home exclusively, eliminating certain foods, eating lesser quantities, substituting meals, taking short fasts, or whatever else – you must make room for eating *with* pleasure and *for* pleasure. Food is something to be enjoyed.

Remember, eating is something you'll probably do for the rest of your life. It is not a fad or an optional chore, it is a marathon exercise to the end. Therefore, you should design a dietary habit that makes you comfortable. There are enough other sources of stress, so aim to minimize the dietary one.

What this means in practice is that you ought to develop a habit of giving yourself permission to treat yourself. Whatever your favorite foods may be, no matter how contrary to all the rules of successful weight-loss, occasionally you must in good conscience, relieve the constraints and indulge unashamedly. So have that scoop of ice-cream, or just relish in a hot-dog, or pamper those taste buds with your heart's desire. After all, when it comes to dietary intake, it is not the food you consume once-in-a-very-long-while that is going to determine your health (or even your weight) status. It is rather the constant daily indulgences, those poor food choices that have the cumulative effect of clogging the arteries, poisoning the liver, destroying the kidneys and increasing girth, while zapping your energy – these are the real determinants.

So many people start out on a new diet, enjoying the results. They're looking good and feeling good. But it only lasts a couple months and then, it's back to the unhealthy eating as usual. They cannot be so 'masochistic' forever. At coffee break, first they itch for some sweet delight that others seem to enjoy, but they would have none of it. Initial discipline to resist is a source of pride and offers protection from the unthinkable, sinful capitulation. They become tense and irritable, later stoic and angry, finally desperate, resigned and eventually indulgent. More often than not, they become recklessly so and indifferent to the consequences. Such people are invariably too hard on themselves – before, during and after the entire futile execise.

You must choose a different course. Cultivate dietary habits that are rational, reasonable and rewarding in terms of both pleasure and weight management.

Do you know what your favorite foods are? Do you have a favorite place to eat? Have you marked special items in the supermarket as yours to enjoy? Then with my permission (and hopefully yours, too) go out and indulge. Just do it. Do it as an exception and not as a general rule. Throw caution to the wind, but not too far into the wind, lest it blow away and soar, leaving you defenseless to face another day.

Pause here, it's a great time for a treat. This one is on me...what are you having?

Commandment #10   Supplement Your Diet

Wise supplementation is a safe, convenient way of obtaining a guaranteed supply of all the essential nutrients that your body needs on a consistent daily basis. It is a complement to a careful diet of normal meals in the real, contemporary world. It is not a substitute for sensible eating, but it acknowledges the problems posed by food technology and personal lifestyle for optimal nutrient intake. It is a modern solution to a modern dilemma.

Millions of North Americans today will consume one or more food supplements in the form of tablets, capsules, powders, oils, solutions and the like. Typically without any prescription, but with their own judgement and common sense they will seek to derive essential food nutrients from such concentrated formulations. Many are derived from natural food sources as extracts or isolates. Some are treated for one reason or another to make stable, convenient, marketable products. Others are essentially prepared by chemical synthesis to molecular specifications. The benefit to the cells of the human body after digestion and assimilation may be different in each case, but the intent is the same.

Supplementation is often touted either as a panacea for all ills or brushed aside as a foolish placebo. It is truly neither. When applied wisely and cautiously, it is rather a scientifically justified means to raise the nutritional status of an individual when there are dietary inadequacies. Clinical research on supplements will continue to give us more conclusive evidence about the role of this unique means of nutritional intervention. It is still a young, empirical science today. It so happens that on this one, the lay public is way out in front of most orthodox professionals who are both unaware and uninterested in the vast reservoir of both consumer experience and clinical responsiveness when put to the test.

Not everyone will agree. On the other side of the coin, there are those who contend that supplementation of the diet is unnecessary, that we will get all our bodies need if we eat a balanced diet. This only begs the question, since the debate then translates to what is a balanced diet in the modern home and who subscribes to it regularly. Nutritionists, educators and others have tried to make the nation eat well, but the forces of opposition, including technology and business, plus advertising and contemporary living, have won the day. Food supplementation has become a convenient and sensible alternative in the real world of fast, convenient, processed and junk foods.

Even when you try to make good food choices, the net value of nutrients you actually get when you eat can often be much reduced or altered with reference to the textbook values. In principle, food processing can seriously affect the nutritive value of the foods that you select from the thousands of supermarket items to construct your three well-balanced daily meals. For example, after early harvesting, transportation, storage, cooking, freezing, canning, over-processing, refining and pasteurization of the food supply, the food value losses are most significantly altered. That's what you take home. Who knows what you eat days later, after you cook it all?

With all this in mind, it is more than just a good idea to supplement your diet with carefully chosen proteins, vitamins and mineral formulation, to ensure that all cellular requirements are met and unavoidable stresses to the body are overcome. You need only think of it as a form of health insurance.

The ideal food supplement that you could choose would be designed to meet established dietary needs. It should do justice to the best scientific knowledge, both by the design of the ingredient deck and the technology of its preparation for maximum stability and bioavailability. The raw material selection must be made with extreme scrutiny to get the best available natural sources of the highest quality. It takes rigorous quality control with state-of-the-art technology to guarantee a minimal deterioration of nutrient value or contamination. Finally, good supplements would be established through careful evaluation and hopefully clinical testing (RCT) to demonstrate their *in vivo* effectiveness.

From what we have learned in this book about cell-defense, about the role of glutathione and about the value of unique whey proteins (**Immunocal™**) to deliver the essential precursor cysteine inside the cell – that is obviously the first order of business in any wise supplementation program. This is the only safe, effective and convenient way to modulate the all-important GSH – nature's prime antioxidant, free radical scavenger and detoxifier inside the cell – and an effective enhancer of the immune system. Regular use of Immunocal™ on a daily basis promises to add life to one's years and maybe even years to one's life.

Other protective vitamin and mineral cofactors also make consummate sense. This might be a good complete vitamin/mineral supplement, or at least one rich in the antioxidants A, C and E, vitamins, together with a couple of B vitamins and antioxidant trace minerals, selenium and zinc.

Then from what we learned also in terms of coping with anxiety and stress, the natural bioactive casein hydrolysate (**PNT 200**™) will be effective in restoring tranquility as it effectively binds to the benzodiazepine (Valium™) – type receptor in the brain.

As for the important need of the major mineral calcium – one could do no better than obtaining it from the ideal natural source: **Pure Milk Calcium**™. But there's much to be gained from other coping strategies.

COPING STRATEGIES

Wellness is becoming an art. The art of life is balance. The key to a healthy lifestyle is also balance: Eating enough but not too much. Exercising in moderation, to preserve your heart and other muscles and not destroy your joints. Obtaining adequate rest without sleeping your life away. Maintaining a positive attitude without pride or presumption. Living with enough stress to find the joy of productivity without paying the high price of burnout. Putting it all together and keeping it there is a challenge. But what a victory you gain when you win. You will become fully alive!

Meeting the challenge of building good health is all in the choices you make, today and every day. Healthy lifestyle choices lead to enjoyment of the best quality of life available to you and increases the odds that yours will be a long and healthy life. As you work toward a goal of building good health, you must remember that the components of good health are interdependent. No benefit will be derived if you eat nothing but junk food and still try to exercise like a professional athlete. Equally, no amount of good nutrition can substitute for adequate rest. If you detest your job, or your spouse, or the weather - no amount of vitamins will convert you into that buoyant, excited extrovert that you aspire to be. If you prove to be a driven workaholic with or without success, you could be just as intense about racquetball and go without sleep or regular meals, only to become a forgotten statistic.

Let's explore four common but often neglected coping strategies that together you will discover can afford an experience of life's best. It's the **R.E.A.L.** thing.

Rest

We choose to begin from a state of Rest.

Many of us may recall as children pouting, whining, throwing tantrums or even begging our parents to allow us to stay up, just for one more hour. We weren't sleepy and our favorite show on TV (or Radio for the oldsters) wasn't over yet. Regardless, we always ended up being sent to bed. Our parents knew what we did not appreciate then: adequate and efficient rest is vital to health. Nothing refreshes the body and mind quite like a good night's sleep, or sometimes a short change of pace in the middle of the day, or even just a few quiet moments to let off steam.

All day long, the body must perform hundreds of functions under a variety of conditions. The routines of just standing, sitting, bending, stretching and walking are not as effortless as they may seem. They require a complex series of muscular movements that gradually exhaust our energy supply. Thinking, too, requires physical energy and even if our work is sedentary but calls for day-long, involved thought processes, we still require physical rest. Moreover, the autonomic nervous system (a biological computer network that keeps us breathing and our heart beating without going anywhere or even having to think about it) must function twenty four hours a day, for the rest of our lives. It too, needs the physiological change provided by efficient rest and sleep. This affords maintenance and restoration.

In fact, in recent years we have learned something about the body clock. We all have a natural circadian rhythm, oscillating on approximately twenty five hour cycles. This spontaneous rhythm regulates a thousand and one biological activities every moment of the day through neurotransmission and hormone secretions, which rise and fall at approximately the same time to determine our body temperature, respiration, mood, degree of alertness and so on. No wonder that most people are "day" folks with maximum performance in the morning when our temperature is normally at a peak. That's when we pump more adrenaline and burn up tissue. Then at night we rest to "cool the pace" and repair (and renew) the machine while we sleep.

In this "instant and plastic" society we are given to immediate, convenient substitutes. So when the body demands rest, many choose caffeine, nicotine and/or alcohol, especially when even at a late hour they are too tense, too keyed up to even think of falling asleep. Many fail to realize that *alcohol* induces sleep, but it interferes with rest; *caffeine* stimulates alertness, but it interferes with concentration; *nicotine* calms the nerves, but it interferes with oxygen requirements for energy; *Valium*™ may induce sleep, but it is addictive. There are no substitutes for sleep.

Adequate rest is more than just sleep. It makes sense often to "take five" sometime in the peak of daily pressure, whether at midmorning after the kids are gone and the chores are complete, or in the middle of the afternoon when the tension of business is at break point or the laboring hands and feet are exhausted. This is an extremely important release valve. It should involve stopping the busy, hectic schedule to change gear consciously, relaxing your muscles and nerves to discover the magical, restoring power of resting for a brief five to ten minutes. It might provide the pick-up needed to fight the common, late-afternoon fatigue. It will relieve much *anxiety*.

Every creative and productive person at some time has felt burnt out, lost or just dead in the water. It's in all great biographies – sometimes with weeks or months of great confusion or depression accompanying plain exhaustion. The key is to see it coming. To stop driving so hard around the curve. To take a break and rest awhile. To get more sleep. To drink less coffee and booze. To take a holiday. To recharge yourself long before the battery goes dead.

Get more rest – it's one coping strategy, necessary but not sufficient.

Exercise

We cannot live in a state of rest. We must move on.

Every one of us needs exercise, today and everyday. The link between exercise and health is well-documented. Most significantly, exercise results in increased intake of oxygen to the cells, improving their ability to function. Such aerobic respiration and the cardiovascular conditioning pay big dividends in health. That saves lives. Even with respect to nutrition, exercise stimulates a healthy appetite, and then helps the cells involved in nutrient digestion and absorption function more efficiently, so that we can get the most from our food and have increased protection from future digestive problems.

That's not all. Exercise affords many more benefits that we are learning to appreciate more and more in this age of Wellness. To mention just some of them:

- Improved mental state (exercise is a *natural tranquilizer*)
- A reduction in the loss of lean muscle mass that normally comes with aging
- An improvement in the heart's collateral circulation and its ability to function
- An increase in the protective HDL cholesterol
- Increased bone density to reduce osteoporosis risk
- Increased mobility of joints that spares increasing morbidity
- An overall improvement in blood circulation, tissue detoxification and mental alertness

Paradoxically, exercise demands energy, yet at the same time, through exercise we derive a big payoff – more energy! Energy is exciting; it is vitality and vigor that translates into a new you. A study at the U.S. National Aeronautics and Space Administration put more than 200 Federal employees on a not-too-strenuous, regular exercise regimen and came up with some truly fascinating health implications. Ninety percent of the participants reported they'd never felt in better health and they had greater stamina; over sixty percent lost weight; almost half of them admitted they felt less strain and tension, they worked harder mentally and physically, enjoyed their jobs more and found their work routines less boring; and almost a third said they slept better.

Such results are being repeated in leading companies all over the world. The Japanese are famous for their work-outs on the shop floor before the morning shift …a definite factor in their remarkable productivity. The Chinese attribute their not infrequent longevity to their simple daily practice of *Tai Chi* exercises. Ordinary people from all walks of life are finding this simple key to better health and a better life -energy through exercise. But despite the fitness craze and participaction programs, more people *watch* and *talk* and *plan* when it comes to exercise, than those who actually *do* exercise. Only you must know your own existing level of exercise and your condition of personal fitness.

Whatever the mechanism of its effect, the results are the same. During exercise you consume more oxygen to produce more energy by aerobic respiration in the cells of your body. With training, the increased blood volume and hemoglobin levels improve the delivery of oxygen. The contractility of your heart becomes more efficient and effective. Your lymphatic drainage is cleared. Your cells' biochemical machinery is "revved up" (increased base metabolic rate) and fat is consumed, leaving stored glycogen in reserve for when you need it most.

Then there is the big bonus for the way you feel as the endogenous hormones, endorphins and enkephalins (related to the opiod narcotics in their physiological function in the brain) become elevated to stimulate that natural high. This is an antidote to depression, a relief to *anxiety*, a booster to self-image and mental outlook, and a spur to self-discipline, motivation and self-determination. You get all of that and more, through exercise. It's a coping strategy *par excellence*.

Rest. Exercise ... now coping strategy # 3: attitude.

Attitude

Exercise is good for the body and produces physical energy. But the human mind itself is the most critical source of all human energy. Our thought processes dominate our metabolic activity, support our immune system, affect our threshold and tolerance to pain, create our daily solutions to life's problems, and on and on. A precious gift, indeed. But, unlike the bumblebee who cannot think about the scientific equations that disprove his ability to fly against all odds, we humans know both our possibilities *and* our limitations. We see the needlework patterns of life on both sides – the mosaic on one side and the tangled mess on the other. We choose the side on which to focus.

Our choice turns-on creativity through our own burning desires. We can experience an abundance of energy and vitality as classical Type A or B personalities. It is not the activity but the attitude that really counts. Negative attitudes produce *anxiety*. They leave us listless and uncreative, agonizing over what to do and what not to do; what may happen or whay may not happen; finally never getting around to doing anything. Instead of steering our lives, we seem to be steered by life. It is an elusive drain of human energy and potential. But positive attitudes turn-on both the body and mind to peak performance. Efficiency is optimized. Resilience is maximized.

The relationship between mental outlook and the immune system is a new active area of research. For a long time it has been known that much of the illness seen daily in doctors' offices and on hospital wards is psychosomatic in origin. The very things we fear often come upon us – whether it be losing our health, our home, or our spouse. Our minds, or rather our thoughts are hurting us! The only way to fight the problem is by changing our attitude ... drugs cannot do it; proper nutrition cannot do it. Using the power of the human mind, we must do it for ourselves. We must develop a positive attitude.

Of course, you remember what it is like to do an activity that you enjoy. If you love skiing, the following scenario may be familiar to you. Regardless of what you did the night before, you get up at four a.m. on a cold morning, have a hearty breakfast at that early hour, burst through the door into the wintry air and do so happily. You are self-motivated. Your self-image is good. You are alive!

On the flip side of the coin, imagine that your proverbial mother-in-law (of whom you may or may not be very fond) is coming for a visit. You struggle to get up early to clean the house and prepare for dinner. You end up literally dragging yourself from bed with the sheets feeling like lead, complaining to yourself all the way. You are *anxious* throughout the day. You are then less than fully alive. But it's all in your mind, nothing else has changed.

True, some tasks are more fun than others. And naturally, you will not typically feel the same degree of enthusiasm for your mother-in-law's visit as for a ski trip. However, a positive attitude and a lifestyle that adheres to this ideal will help keep you in a state of good health, most of the time. The choice is yours, despite the circumstances. Adopting a positive attitude in the face of every situation is clearly a coping strategy that you can ill afford to miss. Otherwise, you will bear a burden of *anxiety* and depressed mood. But you can indeed control your attitude and your thoughts, and thereby control your life.

Life

This is the final component of the R.E.A.L. thing. Rest. Exercise. Attitude. Life. The ultimate goal of any Wellness philosophy or lifestyle is to experience the most of life, the best of life that is possible.

It is experiencing each and every day, the joy of being *alive*. Beyond mere existence and the routine motions and chores of daily activity we all want to discover life. We want to enjoy a life of purpose and fulfillment -- one free from unnecessary *anxiety* and inordinate stress. The inevitable bad day would then be only just a day in the context of a real good life.

Life becomes difficult (though not impossible) in the absence of a healthy body *and* a healthy mind. In all its components and compartments, we infuse value, meaning and enjoyment when we have abundant energy, vitality and peace of mind. This is an asset we can ill afford to lose, so we should do everything to defend the body and calm the mind (as we explored in Parts Two and Three of this book respectively).

As a strategy, the art of living is to learn to seize the moment. We can do without the pain and guilt of the past and certainly without the *anxiety* of the future. We need to recognize as someone else has said:

> Yesterday is history,
> Tomorrow is mystery, but
> Today is a gift –
> That's why we call it *the present*!

Today is life's only present. We seize it, unwrap it and enjoy it, here and now, or we have nothing.

So live today as if it were your last ... and as you do, take advantage of the harvested miracle ingredients from **NATURE'S GOLDMINE**.

Take advantage of the best of *Nature* and the best of *Science* and so ... may you enjoy the best of *Health*.
God bless ...

GENERAL REFERENCES
for further reading

Chapter 1

Jellin JM, Batz F., Hitchen K.,
Natural Medicines Comprehensive Database, (2nd Edition), Published by Therapeutic Research Faculty, Stockton, Ca 1999.

Your Guide To Complementary Medicine, Credit LP, Hartunian SG, Nowak MJ, Avery Publishing Group, New York, 1998

Health Inform's Resource Guide to Alternative Health, Edited by Gotkin J, Page K, Copyright 1997 by Health Inform

Chapter 2

Milk The Deadly Poison, Cohen R., Argus Publishing Inc., Eaglewood Cliffs, New Jersey, 1998

Don't Drink Your Milk, Oski FA MD, Teach Services, 1996

Homogenized Milk may cause your Heart Attack – The XO Factor, Kurt A., Oster MD, Park City Press, 1983

The Face on the Milk Carton, Cooney CB, Doubleday, 1996

Got Milk: The Book, Manning J., Prima Publ., 1999

Chapter 3

Cancer: Cause, Cure and Cover-Up, Godanski R, Nadex Publishing, 2000

The Politics of Cancer Re-visited, Epstein SS, East Ridge Press 1998

The Cancer Conspiracy, Moelaert JJ, Vancouver, BC 1999

The Cure for all Cancers, Clark H., New Century Press, 1993

Chapter 4

Immunology, A Short Course, Benjamin E, Sunshine G, Leskowitz, S, Wiley-Liss, NY, Publishers, 3rd Edit 1996

Immunology, Understanding the Immune System, Elgert KD, Wiley-Liss, NY, Publishers, 1996

GENERAL REFERENCES
for further reading

Chapter 5

Breakthrough In Cell-Defense, Somersall AC, Bounous G, GOLDENeight Publishers, 1999

Chapter 6

Glutathione GSH, Your Body's most powerful healing agent, Gutman J, Schettini S, G & S Health Books Publishers, 2000

Chapter 7

US Surgeon General's Report on Mental Health, 2000

Chapter 8

Principles of Medical Pharmacology, Edited by Kalant H, Roschlan WHE, Sellers EM, University of Toronto Press, 4th Edit, 1985

Chapter 9

Principles of Neuropsycho-pharmacology, Fedman RS, Meyer JS, Quenzer LF, Published by Sinaner, 1997

Overview on Milk Protein-derived Peptides, Hans Meisel, Int. Dairy Journal (1998), 363-373

Physiological Effects of Milk Protein Components, Daniel Torne and Haja Debabbi, Int. Dairy Journal (1998), 383-393

Milk-Borne Bioactive Peptides, Schanbacher FL et al., Int. Dairy Journal (1998)

Chapter 10

Calcium Counts, Annette B, Heslin, JA, Pocket Books, 2000

The Osteoporosis Solution, Germano C, William, MC, Turner L, Kensington Publ. Corp., 2000

Chapter 11

See local Dairy Farmer's Associations Publications

Chapter 12

Your Very Good Health – 101 Healthy Lifestyle Choices, Somersall AC, Harmony With Nature Publishers, 1987

Modern Nutrition in Health and Disease, Edited by Shils M et al., Published by Lippincott, Williams & Wilkins, IXth Edit, 1999

INDEX

INDEX

INDEX

INDEX

INDEX

Ordering Information:

Nature's Goldmine

Single copies.......................$ 19.95US / $24.95CDN
10 or more copies:............. 10% discount

Shipping & handling: $4.00 per single copy

VISA/Mastercard orders:
24-hour Voice Mail
1-800-501-8516
E-Mail: www.goldeneightbooks@aol.com

Or mail your order to:

GOLDENeight Publishers
2-3415 Dixie Road, Unit: 538
Mississauga, Ontario CANADA
L4Y 2B1

Offices also in Atlanta, Georgia USA

Please allow six weeks for delivery